Acne

Proven Natural Remedies for Acne-free Skin

(Learn About the Most Recent Updated Natural Acne)

Teresa Herrick

Published By **John Kembrey**

Teresa Herrick

All Rights Reserved

Acne: Proven Natural Remedies for Acne-free Skin (Learn About the Most Recent Updated Natural Acne)

ISBN 978-1-77485-505-8

No part of this guidebook shall be reproduced in any form without permission in writing from the publisher except in the case of brief quotations embodied in critical articles or reviews.

Legal & Disclaimer

The information contained in this ebook is not designed to replace or take the place of any form of medicine or professional medical advice. The information in this ebook has been provided for educational & entertainment purposes only.

The information contained in this book has been compiled from sources deemed reliable, and it is accurate to the best of the Author's knowledge; however, the Author cannot guarantee its accuracy and validity and cannot be held liable for any errors or omissions. Changes are periodically made to this book. You must consult your doctor or get professional medical advice before using any of the suggested remedies, techniques, or information in this book.

Upon using the information contained in this book, you agree to hold harmless the Author from and against any damages, costs, and expenses, including any legal fees potentially resulting from the application of any of the information provided by this guide. This disclaimer applies to any damages or injury caused by the use and application, whether directly or indirectly, of any advice or information presented, whether for breach of contract, tort, negligence, personal injury, criminal intent, or under any other cause of action.

You agree to accept all risks of using the information presented inside this book. You need to consult a professional medical practitioner in order to ensure you are both able and healthy enough to participate in this program.

Table of Contents

Introduction _____ 1

Chapter 1: What Is Acne _____ 3

Chapter 2: What Is The Reason Do I Suffer From Acne? _____ 6

Chapter 3: Acne And The Mind _____ 14

Chapter 4: Acne And The Gut_____ 24

Chapter 5: Skin Care Products _____ 37

Chapter 6: Acne Scarring And Treatment _ 46

Chapter 7: What To Do Feel Good In Your Own Skin _____ 53

Chapter 8: Acne Action Plan Putting It All Together_____ 61

Chapter 9: My Experiment With Acne Acne 66

Chapter 10: Essential Oils For Natural Skin Care _____ 69

Chapter 11: How To Treat Acne Through Exercise And Stress Reduction _____ 75

Chapter 12: Dietary Tips For Healthful Skin 82

Chapter 13: Lifestyle Improvements To Better Skin Health_____ 87

Chapter 14: A Home Remedies For Acne Recipes _____ 90

Chapter 15: What To Restore Acne Marks And Scars _____ *95*

Chapter 16: Everything About Acne _____ *101*

Chapter 17: Characteristics And Symptoms Of Acne _____ *133*

Conclusion _____ *155*

Introduction

Dear friend,
Acne is an issue that affects many people. I've seen through my own experience how harmful acne can be to your appearance and self-esteem. When I write this article, I am forty-years old. I was plagued by acne throughout my teenage years and into my early 20s. I can remember how awful it made me feel about the appearance of my skin, and also about myself! I determined that I could find a way to get rid of my acne and remain free of acne. It took me a long time and I had to conduct a lot of research. Finally, I discovered the best way to get rid of my acne by using a holistic approach that included the help of my dermatologist and ensuring that my mental, gut well-being and lifestyle contributed to the optimal well-being of my entire body and , consequently, my skin. I do not wish for anyone else to endure the same issues the same amount of time as I did, so this book contains

everything I've learned over the years to ensure that your healing from acne is as fast and painless as you can and last for a long time. In this book, I'm hoping to share the approach I have used to help me and many people overcome the acne. Acne is a complicated issue and has many possibilities for the cause. This book examines how to treat the problem from multiple aspects. It can be used by itself if you suffer from mild acne or wish to take a more natural method to clear acne prior to seeing dermatologists, or is a great supplement to treatments recommended from your dermatologist.

Chapter 1: What Is Acne

Acne symptoms

The medical term used to describe acne vulgaris is. The signs are pustules - an area with a white tip in the centre. Blackheads tiny lumps that are black or yellow in the face, and whiteheads they are similar like blackheads, but they are higher and more white in color. The papules are tiny red lumps beneath the skin, which may be tender or sore. Nodules - massive lumps of hard tissue under the skin that may be painful. Cysts - These are huge lumps that look like boils and are stuffed with pus. Skin that is oily - it is covered in a shiny, oily sebum substance that shows up all day long. Acne scarring can vary from the appearance of red marks to marks that appear on your skin (I will discuss more detail about this issue later in the book).

Acne is most prevalent on the face, but it can also appear on the chest and back.

Who are the people affected?

Acne is more common among teens and young adults. The majority of people affected people are between the ages between 11 and 30. Acne generally disappears when a person grows older and usually before they reach the middle of their twenties. Acne may persist throughout adulthood, approximately 3percent of people older than 35 suffer from acne.

When should you seek medical advice?

If you experience moderate to severe acne , you must schedule an appointment with the GP and they can recommend you to dermatologist. Moderate acne is characterized by the following signs: papules and pustules that have whiteheads and blackheads. Acne that is severe can be characterized by the following signs: pustules, papules, cysts and nodules. It may also cause scarring.

If you suffer from mild acne, you should talk to a pharmacist. they could be able suggest some possible treatments for it. However, in the event that you aren't satisfied with your treatment for any reason, you must consult your GP. The signs of mild acne are oily skin, blackheads, and whiteheads with a few papules as well as pustules.

Treatments for acne could last for around three months before they begin to take effect, so wait and gentle with yourself. If the treatment stops effective after the time period, consult the GP or dermatologist.

Chapter 2: What Is The Reason Do I Suffer From Acne?

What causes Acne

Acne is caused by excessive sebum that is on the skin combining and dead cells of the skin, which result in a blockage inside the hair follicles on the skin. This could lead to whiteheads and blackheads. The bacteria that reside present on the surface of the skin, which is normally harmless , can end up contaminating the hair follicles that are plugged and cause papules, pustules and cysts.

There are a variety of factors which can trigger the excessive sebum to show up over the surface of the body.

1. Hormones

Testosterone

Testosterone is a hormone which naturally increases in boys and girls in their teens. It plays a significant role in the development and growth of both girls and boys. However , excessive levels of testosterone may cause increase in the amount of sebum. Testosterone can also rise when a woman suffers from polycystic ovary syndrome , which often causes acne.

Cortisol

Cortisol is an hormone that is triggered by stress. If your mind is aware of the threat the body produces this hormone in order to prepare for the anxiety. In the case of a situation where you have to flee from something, your body produces cortisol, which blocks the non-essential tasks of your body like digestion of food, in order for the body to get the energy required to escape that threat. But if you are producing cortisol over a lengthy period of time (maybe due to the fact that you're having a rough moment and your mind is constantly thinking about threats to your wellbeing or your life) it may begin to impact your body in negative ways. One thing that could occur can be that the body could increase the amount of sebum produced. Other signs that could result because your body is constantly producing cortisol levels too high are depression, anxiety stomach problems headaches, heart disease sleep issues and weight gain, memory loss and difficulty in concentration.

Progesterone

Progesterone is increased in women about two weeks prior to their period. Progesterone's increased production could cause excessive sebum be produced. It generally calms down once the woman begins her menstrual cycle. Also, it gets more intense when a woman is pregnant. This means that acne can pop out or worsen at these moments.

2. Diet

Although it's a bit controversial although I do believe there is a connection between the food we eat and the condition that our skin is in. I've found through the personal experiences of changing my diet did not just improve my skin, but also enhanced my energy levels and overall well-being. There is some scientific evidence that is now emerging that confirms this.

If you consume foods that have an elevated glycemic index, like refined sugars or starchy foods on a frequent basis, it can increase your blood sugar levels and may result in a rise in insulin, which is believed to trigger excessive sebum. There's also a link between eating cow's milk regularly and acne, because dairy foods are laced with hormones, which can cause skin producing excessive oil and swelling.

I will discuss the relationship between gut health, diet and the acne issue in a subsequent chapter.

3. Stress and mental state

There is a connection between cortisol, the hormone that causes stress, and acne. Stress or anxiety may trigger your body to release this hormone. I believe that the way that you perceive yourself and the way you feel others perceive you is the main cause of anxiety and stress. This could be a reason if you have an acne problem and are self-conscious about it, which can cause more anxiety and stress. Insufficient quality sleep can cause your body to release cortisol. I'll go over the relationship between the brain and skin in a subsequent chapter. In this chapter, I will provide suggestions on how to alter your attitude and decrease the stress and anxiety.

4. Habits and the environment

There is a connection between acne and the cleanliness of your home and your everyday habits. It is essential to ensure the bedding you use is tidy and you change your pillowcase every day since when you sleep, you sweat and scratch your face against the pillow case. It is recommended to wash your pillow case at least every couple of days. It's recommended to purchase more pillow cases, and keep a few extra ones available. It is a good idea to purchase silk pillow covers because they're less rough on the skin, and therefore less likely to cause irritation on the skin. They are excellent for preventing the skin from aging! You can purchase them on Amazon They are slightly more expensive than cotton ones, but I believe your skin will be worth it!

I suggest you wash the other sheets at least twice per week.

If you wear make-up, it is crucial to ensure that you regularly clean your sponges and brushes. I suggest cleaning your sponges each time you use them because they are a great source of bacteria. If possible, do not using a sponge. apply your foundation using fingertips or a foundation brush. Brushes need to be cleaned each once a week. I suggest buying an antibacterial wash-up liquid. It's inexpensive and works effectively. When you do not wash your brushes you can apply alcohol to the bristles on the brush. This will kill any bacteria. You can buy pure alcohol at Amazon or any pharmacy or chemist. You can decant it in an empty plastic spray bottle. ensure that you label it, and make sure it is out of reach of children.

When you wash your face, whenever possible, it's ideal to dry it with a facial towel intended meant for use by you only. It is a good idea to purchase a face towel for each single day. They're not expensive, and you can use them every day, and clean them out at after the duration of the week.

Although they don't cause acne by themselves but they could contribute to making it worse.

Acne myths

Squeezing out spots and blackheads is the most effective way to eliminate acne. However, this is a myth , and If you keep squeezing spots and blackheads it can aggravate your skinand make the signs worse, and even cause the formation of scars.

Sunbathing and sunbeds may help in reducing acne. However, there is no evidence that suggests it's not possible to. I was a sunbed user in my younger years because of this reason however, I didn't notice any significant changes. The risk of developing sunburn and early aging due to sunbeds are far greater than the benefits they could have on acne. If you decide to spend time in the sun, ensure you're wearing an eye-shade of at minimum factor 50, and an additional sunblock for the body. A final note to be aware of sunbeds and sunbathing is that they can very quickly result in permanent pigmentation marks to the skin, especially in the case of acne medications.

Acne is contagious - Acne isn't infectious and you can't transmit it to anyone else.

Chapter 3: Acne And The Mind

The skin and mind connection

As we have discussed previously, in the past, cortisol is a stress-related hormone and has been identified as one of the primary causes of acne. My opinion is that today's stress and anxiety is at an all-time level! There is so many demands on each of us to conform and behave in a certain manner and to achieve certain outcomes after a certain point in time. We must conform to the norm and, often, suppress our true emotions. For instance, if are a woman, it's just not acceptable socially to be angry , therefore we must suppress our emotions. The same is true for males. It's not appropriate in the society for them to be crying and they must be strong instead. The inability to express our feelings and thinking that we must do more, appear like a certain manner and be more to fit in a small mold in the society is extremely stressful! If you're suffering from acne, you could add another stress factor on your to-do list!

So how do we deal with all the stressors? The best way is to do our best to ensure that we receive the approval of other people. What happens if, after all the hard work we are still not up to the Instagram standards of living or what happens if we live an excellent life according to our standards, and somebody says that it's not enough?

Can I suggest a different option? Do you love yourself? Perhaps we don't need to be a part of the society. Maybe we can choose our own way and achieve satisfaction and happiness by ourselves, with no approval from other people. In the end, how miserable would it be were able to enjoy the support of all those around us, and yet we were unhappy and discontent? More than ever, I believe we have to find our way through life to ensure that we feel satisfied and not overly concerned about what the society thinks. This may require some serious internal work and takes time but I believe it's worth considering what you want out of life, and then focusing your efforts towards making that occur instead of trying to fit in with the social norms. It is my belief that when we take this approach, many of the stress and stress we feel will eventually disappear. There are a few good books I would suggest for those who want to learn more about how you can be yourself and grow further. Awaken your Giant Within written by Anthony Robbins, As a Man Thinks By James Allen, I Am Enough by Marissa Peer, Opening the Door of Your Heart by Ajahn Brahm.

There are many factors that could make us feel stressed and I'd recommend finding the root of the issue and getting it in the right place. If you require help, don't be afraid to confess that you are in need of help. Seek help from a trusted person or an expert. I am convinced that healthy mental health can aid in reducing, if not remove pimples (depending on the reason for the acne) as well as there are many other benefits to having a healthy mental state. They include more motivation, better relationships, more self-confidence and a greater ability to focus and accomplish tasks accomplished, feeling generally more content ......and it just is endless.

Depression and Anxiety Caused by Acne

I've learned from my personal experiences that having acne can cause you to feel self-conscious, depressed and stressed! It's just that it always seems to be in your head and you think about what other people are thinking while you're talking to them, and whether they're even taking note of your skin!

There are some actions you can take to alleviate depression and anxiety.

1. Change your perspective - As I am at the age of forty , I have concluded that most people I talk with and have talked to previously tend to think of themselves as well as their personal problems , and do not have the energy or time to know whether we possess clear, smooth skin. It's true that this may not be a good idea because I've experienced how it feels to be a victim of acne and how unpleasant this can affect you, yet it's worthwhile to think

about it and could provide one of the factors to helping you manage being a victim of acne until it goes away.

2. Meditation is a fantastic way to unwind your mind and relax your body. It's simple to perform however it may take several minutes to silence the thoughts of your head. I suggest starting with 5 minutes every day, and increase the amount gradually. There are numerous apps you can download that offer guided meditations. You are also able to find the videos on YouTube. I suggest using guided meditations at minimum in the beginning because it helps you concentrate more. The other advantages of meditation are that it boosts your emotional well-being improves self-awareness and reduces isolation, boosts feelings of self-love and acceptance, increases attention span, may increase compassion, helps combat addictions, improve sleep, eases the pain and may reduce blood pressure. It is definitely worthwhile to make meditation a daily practice, because it will enhance

your overall wellbeing by committing to it for only one or two minutes every day!

3. Yoga This is a good practice to ease the mind and body. It involves executing specific yoga postures that require strength and stability. It also requires deep breathing and paying attention to your breathing. You can take an online yoga class at no cost on YouTube or attend a local yoga class. Yoga's benefits include reducing anxiety and stress, increases flexibility, improved muscle strength and tone, improved breathing and energy levels, reduction in weight, protection against injuries, enhanced circulation and cardio health, aids in improving posture, decreases the blood sugar level, improves the immune system and regulates your adrenal glands in order to reduce cortisol levels. It's definitely worth picking the time to practice this. I would recommend starting with a single class per week, and gradually progressing to three classes.

4. Aerobic exercise is crucial, according to me, for reducing stress, boosting your mood and helping you overcome

depression. Even a brief period of time has been proven to increase your mood. Other benefits include: it enhances sleep, increases brain power, boosts the immune system controls weight, decreases the levels of blood sugar, relieves chronic pain, and reduces blood pressure. There are many types of aerobic exercise, including running, swimming, walking dance, cycling and kickboxing, as well as aerobic classes. I highly recommend adding an aerobic workout in your daily routine. For the beginning, I would suggest 30 minutes three times a week . Then increase the amount until you are comfortable with it.

5. Spending time with people you enjoy is a fantastic option to let go of your thoughts and forget about a particular problem like acne is to be with people you enjoy being around. Engaging in a fun activity with your friends or engaging in an engaging conversation keeps your mind off of you and your worries and allows you to connect to another person. It may sound simple, but it's an integral an integral part of healing and, often, it's

other people who help us navigate through difficult times in our lives.

6. Volunteering and giving Anything that takes your mind away from your self-defeating thoughts about your troubles is a good thing. Studies have proven that helping others by giving improves self-esteem. it also provides you with connections with others and may lead to the making of new acquaintances. The act of giving will allow you to develop as a person, and you'll help others while doing it.

Here are some suggestions to give a hand - think about the things and issues you are passionate about, then locate an organization in your area and determine whether you can help through volunteering or by donating. You can make a donation to national charities that carry out the work you love. There are many ways to give more to your loved ones by giving them either time or listening to their concerns or giving them a cup of coffee. There are many ways to help and you don't need be wealthy in order to be generous, simply discover your own method to give and start with a small amount. As your self-esteem begins to grow, it will become addicting and you'll want to give more!

7. Take care of your acne with a professional - it can trigger mental health problems for all people at any age. If you experience feeling depressed, anxious, or anger for prolonged durations of time or feel like you are being withdrawn from social interactions, it's an appropriate time to seek assistance. There's no excuse not to seek assistance if you are certain there's something wrong. The sooner you address the issue and seek assistance, the more effective. There are professionals who can be contacted, including counsellors. They will assist you in determining what is the issue. There may be a different issue entirely and it's the acne that's creating the issue in the first place. Life coaches can assist you in moving forward and help you plan what you would like to achieve in your life and assist you in achieving it. Therapists - there's many different kinds of

treatments for depression and anxiety which can be performed by a trained therapist who is certified in the field to assist or even eliminate depression and anxiety, for instance treatment with EMDR (Eye movement desensitisation Reprocessing) is a highly efficient therapy for trauma. Hypnotherapy is a different, highly effective method of dealing with anxiety and past trauma. Acupuncture is a wonderful method to relieve and release tension by working on the energy points within the body. EFT (Emotional Freedom Technique) is a kind of counseling that concentrates on your feelings and helps you heal the trauma of your past through the use of energy points. It is based on how you feel personally and if you have any other events or experiences you've experienced that contributed to the anxiety you feel and the personal circumstances you face. The best place to begin is to seek suggestions with your GP.

Chapter 4: Acne And The Gut

There has been a constant debate over the connection to diet as well as acne however , there is now research that has proven a connection with gut health, and wellbeing and health of the other parts of your body, including the skin. The study shows that poor digestive health can trigger acne and other problems like mental health issues, problems with sleep, low energy, chronic fatigue auto immune disorders and weight changes skin irritations, and an upset stomach.

One of the main reasons for poor gut health is a diet that is deficient in vital nutrients and vitamins. It also is filled with refined sugars and refined carbs and processed food items. Additionally, food pairing (the meals we select to eat during the same meal) may play a role.

The standard diet of the UK includes foods that are rich in refined carbs along with refined sugars, alcohol and. We eat convenience food like ready-to-eat meals and takeaway food and aren't aware of the food we are putting in our bodies.

Diet

First, let's take a examine the foods that aren't good for your gut health.

Refined carbohydrates and sugars white bread pasta, pastries, breakfast cereals cakes, cookies sweets, sweetened sodas etc. These foods can fuel the bad bacteria that live inside your gut, and will reduce the number of beneficial bacteria in your gut. When you consume refined carbs or sugars, the insulin and blood sugar levels to increase and when they drop to a lower level, it can trigger a sugar craving. It is then a continuous cycle that could quickly turn into an addiction to sugar! A high intake of refined sugars and carbohydrates frequently consumed can cause inflammation of the gut and the other parts of the body. It can lead to more serious diseases like cancer. It is not possible to find any nutritional benefit in refined carbohydrates , therefore it won't hurt anyone even if we drastically reduce or completely eliminate them out of our daily diet. I suggest that you keep a little bit every now and then is okay because if say to yourself that you will not ever have it again, you'll feel as if you're denying yourself. If you can incorporate this practice into your daily routine, and you might be amazed at how great you feel and the more energy you feel after just several days!

Alcohol makes the stomach create more acid than is needed which causes irritation and causes inflammation of your stomach's lining. It also kills beneficial bacteria and good bacteria that reside in your stomach. In essence, alcohol is poison to your body . It can lead to many issues for your health when it is consumed regularly over a long time. This includes elevated blood pressure and liver diseases, dementia, depression, cancer skin irritations, premature aging and infertility. Reduce or even eliminating it altogether out of your diet is among the most beneficial things you can do to improve your gut health and skin, as well as and overall well-being and overall health.

Processed food - store prepared meals purchased at the store such as sausage, cheese, bacon, crisps, ham salami, canned food pizza, pate, etc.

All of these food items are deficient in fiber and are contain high levels of trans fatsand sodium, and preservatives. These increase cholesterol levels, causes irritation to the gut lining and triggers inflammation. If you consume them regularly for a long time, these foods could cause the following negative effects on the body: obesity, heart disease as well as high blood pressure, and diabetes. If you make a conscious effort to reduce these foods , you'll start to feel better quickly and can avoid developing illnesses in the future.

Cows milk - I have personally observed that dairy from cows can have a negative impact on my skin and digestive tract due to the fact that it causes inflammation and excessive sebum on my skin. But, there are positive benefits of cow's milk and some prefer it. I personally prefer dairy products that are plant-based, such as goat's cheese and goat's milk. I believe that you must discover what works for you in regards to dairy. Keep a diary of your food intake to check if you suffer from any adverse reactions when you consume cow's dairy. If so, it may be worth cutting back or replacing it with goat's milk or alternative plant-based products.

What should I eat to maintain a healthy gut and healthy skin?

Once you've figured out what foods to stay clear of, let's talk about what foods to consume to improve the health of your digestive system and which will help clear your skin.

Green Vegetables: Broccoli as well as courgette, kale, spinach (zucchini) as well as cabbage, Brussel sprouts, etc. These are all high in fiber and help improve the health of the bacteria in your digestive tract, as well as having a high water content and are brimming with vital vitamins and minerals. They should be consumed as it is possible to do so at every meal and form the major portion of your daily diet. There are numerous benefits to eating often over a long duration of time! In the initial few weeks, your digestion will begin to improve and you'll begin to notice improvement on your skin. In the longer term, you'll be able to significantly reduce the risk of suffering from heart cancer, diabetes obesity, high blood pressure.

Other fruits and vegetables - Aubergine (eggplant) peppers and parsnips, carrots, Sweet potato, turnip bananas, avocados, apples and tomatoes, lemons, pears, etc.

They should also constitute a significant portion in your daily diet. They are also high in water, fibre and minerals. However, they have a slight increase in natural sugars and should be consumed less frequently than green vegetables. They have a lot of benefits for health in regular consumption, such as better digestion and gut health and better glucose levels in the blood, an improved feeling of well-being, and more energy and a lower risk of developing heart cancer, diabetes and obesity as well as high blood pressure.

Beans and Legumes : chickpeas and lentils, kidney beans, peas black beans, pinto beans, etc. These food items are a fantastic source of fiber, protein and vitamins as well as minerals and vitamins. If consumed regularly, they can improve digestive health, assist in control blood sugar levels, and increase cholesterol levels.

Whole Grains - Brown Rice Whole wheat bread barley, oatmeal, quinoa and whole wheat pasta. These are foods that are rich in fiber, which helps maintain a healthy digestion and improve the health of your gut.

Meat , fish, and eggs Chicken, fish lamb and beef (all non-processed) These food items contain significant levels of protein. Protein is vital to building and maintain the muscle mass, bone cartilage skin and blood. It is also utilized by the body to create hormones and enzymes. Choose healthy organic meat that is lean and natural. Protein can be obtained from different sources like legumes and beans, thus there is no need to add meat to your diet if you don't currently consume meat.

Fermented foods include sauerkraut, apple cider vinegar and kimchi, as well as cultured yoghurt and more. These are foods that contain probiotics, which are vital for improving gut healthand immune system, and aid in weight loss. These foods are simple to add to your diet and offer many health benefits.

Water - It's so vital to drink plenty of water to maintain your gut and general health. It aids in the elimination of out toxins in your body and balance blood sugar levels, keep joints and muscles working. Personally, I've noticed changes in clarity and firmness my complexion when I consume the correct amount of water as opposed to those who do not. I understand that if drink sparkling pop, water might be boring, but if eliminate the pop and substitute it with water, you'll see a drastic increase on your levels of energy as well as general health and wellbeing and also your skin. After you've switched to water, it'll only take some time to begin to get used to the flavor of water and appreciate the benefits it brings for your body. It is recommended to drink 2 liters of water each daily.

A balanced diet , including all the mentioned foods in the following order can drastically enhance the overall health and wellbeing of your digestive system and consequently your skin.

50 % green vegetables. 20 percent other vegetables. 10% of fermented food items.

20% of one or both of the following: legumes and beans, or whole grains, eggs, fish, meat and eggs.

Foods that are a combination

Food combing can enhance your digestion and the health of your digestive tract. A few studies have revealed that it's harder for the digestive system to process certain foods when they are consumed together as different kinds of food require different time to digest and require different digestive enzymes in order to digest them. The fundamental rules for food combining is to consume fruits on empty stomachs, and don't consume protein or starches (potatoes bread, potatoes etc.) during the same meal and make sure you don't drink fluids for 30 minutes prior to and after meals. Certain people adhere to the concept of the concept of combining food and notice huge differences, but others experience only a slight difference. If you suffer from poor digestion, it's worth trying this method and see whether it can help you.

Probiotics

Probiotics are microorganisms which provide positive health benefits to your gut. They reduce bad bacteria, and increase the good bacteria that reside in your gut . They reduce the inflammation that is positive for skin. They are naturally found in food items like cultured yoghurt and sauerkraut. They can also be found in kefir, sauerkraut miso, tempeh and Kimchi. You can also purchase probiotic supplements. I suggest taking a probiotic supplement each day. It's not a bad idea to consume certain foods listed in the previous paragraphs as well. If you're sensitive to dairy products, you should stay away from yogurt.

What should you be looking for in a great probiotic supplement?

The first step is to be sure to review the label. The probiotic is made up of live bacteria. The recommended daily dosage is between 1 and 10-billion live microbes which means that they need to be properly stored and consumed prior to the expiration date. The two most popular probiotic strains comprise Lactobacillus as well as Bifidobacterium. These strains include L. Acidophilus, L. Casei, L. Plantarum, B. Lactis, B. Longum, B. Bifidum. Both strains are suggested improve your gut health to reduce acne.

Other Supplements to Clear Acne

There are numerous supplements that help remove acne. Like I said in the previous article, anything that could have an anti-inflammatory impact on the body can help remove acne. For that reason, I would recommend the below supplements.

Zinc It has anti-inflammatory properties that help to accelerate the healing process. It is often utilized in treating acne. Vitamin D is known to have anti-inflammatory properties as well as antimicrobial qualities (these are able to help fight the overgrowth of bacteria). Vitamin D supplements are advised for those who spend a significant amount of time inside and/or don't live in a warm climate. If you reside in a climate that is sunny and spend a substantial amount of time outdoors , it is unlikely that you need to use supplements with vitamin D since you will get vitamin D from sun via your skin.

B complex vitamins help the body to create healthy skin cells. They also reduce inflammation and may aid in reducing how much sebum the skin produces.

A supplement with one of the B vitamins is great for acne.

B1 - Thiamin

B2 - Riboflavin

B3 - niacin

B5 is pantothenic acid.

B6 - pyridoxine

B7 Biotin

B9 - Folic acid

B12 - cobalamin

Vitamin A is a vitamin that helps improve cell growth and healing of the skin and is also anti-inflammatory and is an antioxidant (prevents cell damage caused through free radicals). Be aware that you may have been given vitamin A in a form or another by your physician, if that is the case, you should not consume any vitamin A supplement.

Vitamin C is a potent antioxidantthat assists in speeding the healing process and is extremely anti-inflammatory.

Vitamin E can help improve your immune system It also reduces inflammation and increases cell growth.

Vitex Angus Cactus -it helps to balance hormones and is especially helpful during the period. it is also anti-inflammatory.

Turmeric is a powerful anti-inflammatory. it's antibacterial, helps to speed up healing, it enhances brain function, and it is a potent antioxidant.

Be sure to consult with your physician before taking one of the supplements. Also, be sure to not exceed the dosage recommended by your doctor.

Chapter 5: Skin Care Products

Making a routine for skin care

The following tips may be counterintuitive, but trust me when I say it is logical ......

Avoid using drugstore products specifically designed for acne that contain harsh ingredients like alcohol. These products are made to cause dry skin.

Although it might help you feel better right away after applying the product and your skin could appear clean, you'll be able to tell that it won't last for very long. This is because you've removed your skin of its natural oils. It must exert twice as much effort to replace these oils, which means it will produce more oil in order to help compensate!

If you suffer from acne that is active You must maintain a simple routine for your skincare routine and gentle, so that you wash thoroughly the skin, but don't aggravate the acne. It is also important not to dry out and cause skin irritation. It's worthwhile to invest the most money you can to purchase top quality products.

The next routine should be carried out in the both in the morning and evening. Only apply SPF the first thing in the morning.

Cleanse

The way you cleanse your skin is vital. Doing it the right manner is crucial. The aim is to get rid of any makeup or impurities off your skin in the gentlest method possible. Step 1: Remove your makeup first. To take off any eye makeup. I suggest applying a gentle makeup remover, one that doesn't contain alcohol to get rid of the eye makeup. A makeup remover for eyelashes that is oil-based can help remove mascara and completely remove eye makeup. Step 2: Take off all of your makeup. The most effective cleanser to get rid of the makeup you have is cleansing balm , or cleansing oil. Although it seems counterintuitive to apply oil on a skin that is oily but the oil contained in the cleanser is the best method of breaking down the makeup and eliminate the excess oil from your face without stripping the skin and will not cause more oils to the skin. Step 3: Once you've removed your makeup, cleanse your face using an easy, non-foaming cleanser with a low pH and read the label to ensure that it is the product you are buying. I would suggest using a cleanser that is washed off and contains the oil of tea trees. The oil tea tree is an excellent natural ingredient for treating acne as it's anti-inflammatory, antiseptic and helps heal wounds, soothes and anti fungal. It also cleanses thoroughly.

Tone

Toning can help balance and soothe the skin. get rid of excess oil and even the pH on your skin. It is crucial to choose a toner without alcohol that's gentle for the skin. Also, I suggest using a toner with the oil of tea trees. Apply the toner to the cotton pad and then apply it to the skin. Don't apply it to the skin since this can pull and pull the skin, causing unnecessary irritation and stress. Dry the toner and proceed onto the next stage.

Moisturise

The purpose of moisturizing the skin is to ensure that the barrier of your skin is in good health, and to soothe the skin and maintain the level of moisture in balance. It is vital to moisturize your skin when you suffer from acne to ensure that your skin's health levels are maintained and the sebaceous glands don't have to overwork to produce more oil in order to boost the moisture levels up. If your skin is becoming dry, although it might appear like you're drying the acne at first, it's not because in the end, your skin will need produce more oil in order to compensate , and you'll return to the beginning. When selecting a moisturiser, make sure you choose an oil-free lighter gel or lotion that is non-comedogenic. . If possible, use fragrance-free with ingredients that are soothing, like glycerine, demethicone, hyaluronic acids and. These ingredients help to lock in moisture into the skin, without clogging pores. Also, ensure that you read the label. Apply the moisturiser using a gentle applying it to the neck and face.

Sun protection

It may appear like an extra expense, however this isn't an alternative! No matter what your skin type and no matter where you reside, it's essential to apply SPF on your face prior to heading out. Your face is always exposed to the elements, and it's not long before this affects the skin by becoming more sensitive, leading to premature aging and in certain cases, skin cancer.

When selecting the best SPF ensure that it is an incredibly light formula, such as lotion, and ensure that it's SPF percentage is at or near 50. Apply it as the final phase of your regular routine of skincare by gently rubbing a generous amount on your neck and face.

There are other actions that could be added between two and three times per week.

Exfoliate

Exfoliating is the process of removing dead skin cells off the skin's surface thus helping keep the pores free of harmful germs and skin cells that have died accumulation. There are two kinds of exfoliation, the physical one - which are usually made up of facial scrubs, and they are done by rub them on the skin in order to eliminate old skin cells. The second kind is chemical and comes available in gel or liquid formulas that are sprayed on the skin, and washed off after a particular period of time (usually between 10 and twenty minutes). Physical exfoliators aren't suitable for acne as the friction created when you rub the product on the face could cause irritation to the skin and cause breakout to worsen. Chemical exfoliators are the best choice for acne as they accomplish their job by eating away at dead skin cells, without causing irritation or inflammation to the skin. When you are choosing an exfoliator, check for the following ingredients: glycolic acid, salicylic acid and/or lactic acids. It is crucial to speak with your dermatologist prior to deciding to introduce an exfoliator into your regimen because you might already be taking an approved treatment for acne that can exfoliate your skin.

Masks for faces

Masks for face can be utilized as an additional treatment for the skin. The most effective type of face mask to use for acne concerns is an easy face mask that is soothing, cleansing and moisturizing. It must contain components like camomile that soothe, salicylic acid to cleanse and expel impurities, and a moisturizing ingredient like honey or the hyaluronic acid. It is essential to not choose an exfoliation mask that is harsh and drying. It's a good idea to test masks and exfoliators to see how they impact your skin. Use them only once per week for the first time and, as long as they're not drying your skin, then you can increase the frequency up to 2 to 3 every week.

Skin Care Products that Target Acne

On-the-spot treatments

These are usually the form of gels that can be applied directly on the surface to dry it. They are made up of ingredients like saltylic acid and tea tree oils. They should be applied to the site only and should not be applied to the entire skin. They can help dry out the area and help speed up healing.

Retinoids

Retinoids come in various forms including over-the-counter and prescription only. If you're seeing an dermatologist, they will decide the basis of whether they believe you'll be benefited and prescribe in accordance with. Retinoids which can be prescription by a dermatologist include retina or tretinoin. It is usually as gel or cream and Accutane that comes with pills. The retinoids that are available on the market comprise retinol in different forms, and they are available with gels and creams. Retinoids have a beneficial effect on acne. the creams and gels are effective in removing dead skin cells from the surface of your skin, preventing them from growing up and blocking hair follicles. Accutane reduces Sebum created by your skin and thereby decreasing the chance of your pores becoming blocked. It is vital to apply a sunblock while applying the retinoids.

As a side note, If you are able you can, avoid rubbing your areas. I understand how tempting it is, but it may cause scarring on the skin as it weakens the collagen in the area. If you must squeeze a bump, then ensure the spot has the appearance of a white or yellow head. If you attempt at squeezing a lump into the skin, it will not explode and cause skin irritation.

Methods for safely squeezing an area: First clean the area thoroughly and then wrap a towel between your fingers that you'll use. Apply pressure to the sides of the spot until pus is released from the top. Then, apply an antiseptic solution to stop bacteria from entering the skin. If it's swelling and red, then the best option is to use a compress cold to achieve an anti-inflammatory impact.

Chapter 6: Acne Scarring And Treatment

One of the unavoidable adverse effects of acne may be the appearance of acne scarring. There are various kinds of scarring and various methods to enhance the appearance of scarring or eliminate it completely.

Different types of Acne Scars

Discoloration - they are usually brown or red marks that are left behind after the area heals on your skin.

Scars that have been raised - they are usually found on the back and chest and can be seen above the skin.

Atrophic scars are the areas where the skin is compressed. They come in a variety of forms - ice pick scars have a V-shaped, while box scars are more broader U-shaped scars.

The treatment for Acne Scars

It is always advisable to speak with your dermatologist, and they can suggest a treatment plan for you. It is only possible to begin treatments for scars from acne when the acne is treated successfully and has stopped appearing. If you're experiencing mild scarring (just some discoloration) then you'll be able treat this at home using topical treatments. If you are suffering from more severe the scarring (depressed and raised scars) it will have to be treated in the clinic.

Treatment at Home

There are many products available at home to combat acne scarring.

Products that contain the ingredient retinol (Retinoids) There are a variety of products with this ingredient. It is usually used in the event that you've experienced acne or have an oily or mixed skin type. I suggest the use of a serum or lotion that contains Retinol instead of a thick cream because the cream could be too heavy and oily for the skin and may block your pores once more.

The benefits of retinol include that it assists the skin produce more collagen and recover faster, it can smooth the skin and improve circulation, thus improving the color of your skin.

Products that contain vitamin C I would suggest using a lotion or serum rather than cream. Its benefits include that it aids the skin produce more collagen, it improves the appearance and improves the appearance of skin.

Products that contain salicylic acid Avoid any creams with a heavy texture and opt to lighter formulations. Its benefits are that it exfoliates your skin and cleanses the pores, cleansing the skin, giving it a clearer and more radiant. This is particularly beneficial for those with an oily skin due to the purifying effect on the skin.

Glycolic acid is a component of many products can result in brighter skin, clearer and more radiant, as well as exfoliating and eliminating discolouration and aid in reducing the appearance of lines and wrinkles.

In the end, I'd suggest using one of the products listed above to determine the outcomes you can expect and if it's suitable for your skin. There are times when some of these products are too harsh for some types of skin, so it's essential to test it out and keep an eye on your skin. If the product is irritating your skin or you're not seeing any difference, you should try other products.

A clinic for treatment

There are many highly effective treatments you can receive at a medical clinic to treat the more severe forms of scarring. Be sure to do your homework prior to visiting any clinic, and look for reviews and recommendations. Consult your dermatologist about the best treatment for you and a good treatment to seek.

Resurfacing with lasers

There are various kinds of lasers that are used to rejuvenate skin. Erbium Yag - This is a less intense treatment that is suitable for scarring with less. Fraxel - This is a more thorough treatment that only concentrates on the area being treated. CO2RE is utilized more specifically on the skin's surface or deeper to address deeper skin pigmentation and scars. skin. Lasers function by producing thermal energy that is absorbed by the skin. They then vaporize the damaged skin, and also stimulate new collagen production to help revitalize the skin.

The treatment doesn't require a lot of in terms of downtime and you'll be able to generally return to work or to your normal routine within a couple of days. It is possible to experience redness and peeling for a few days following the treatment. The price can vary from PS800 up to PS1,900 per treatment. Typically, you will require 3 to six treatments.

Avoid sun exposure and be sure to wear an SPF at least factor 50 following the treatment.

The results are long-lasting.

Micro needling

The procedure involves pricking the skin using tiny needles. This is a controlled injury and after it heals, the skin starts producing more collagen which in turn increases the size of the skin. This procedure can be carried out in a beauty or clinic salon, but must be done by a certified professional. It is ideal for moderate to light scarring. Your skin could appear flaky and red during the first few days after. Avoid sun exposure and ensure that you apply an SPF of at least 50 after getting the procedure.

The price ranges from PS100 to PS300 per single session typically, you'll get three to 6 treatments.

Chemical peels

There are three different qualities of chemical peels, medium, superficial and deep. It will depend on how severe your scarring is which one to pick. They function by exfoliating and taking off the top layer of skin and reveal, which smothers the skin beneath. The more extensive peels can be risky.

It could cost between PS60 between PS100 for mild peels, and up to PS500 for more intense peels. If you have the deeper peels, generally, you only have one treatment , while with milder peels you'll usually get a series of three to six treatments. When you have mild or moderate peels you may experience peeling and redness that lasts over a period of a couple days or weeks. The results aren't permanent, and you'll have to keep the results going through additional treatments. If you have a deeper peel, you may experience swelling that can last for between 2 and 2 weeks. You may also experience itching for up to two months. The effects are long-lasting.

Chapter 7: What To Do Feel Good In Your Own Skin

There are numerous things are possible to do in order to feel more comfortable and enhance look of skin right away.

Makeup

Makeup can soften and alter the appearance of acne while making you feel more confident about how you appear.

If you are using an excellent non-comedogenic foundation, it's okay to apply makeup to acne. Be sure to remove it immediately after you're at the ease of your home, allowing the skin breath.

Foundation and concealer

If you are applying makeup, begin with foundation. Be sure you match the color to your neck, not the shade of your face because the skin might have a different colour (especially in the case of acne). Use a light layer over your face, and blend into the hairline along the neck. You only want to even the complexion at this point. Do not be concerned if you detect spots. It's better to use your fingertips instead of the foundation brush or sponge since brushes and sponges can contain bacteria. Then, apply concealer (choose one with an extremely thick consistency because it provides complete coverage). The concealer should be the same shade of your foundation, however it should have a slight yellow hue to help counteract the redness on the area. Apply it using a tiny brush for concealer, but make sure that you thoroughly wash the brush first with alcohol. Begin by applying it to the center of the spot and blend it on the rest of the face using gentle strokes of feathers. Be sure to be careful with your concealer and foundation because it will only bring out the acne and make your skin appear cakey if applied too much. The objective is to smooth out your skin tone , making the acne less apparent, but not to make an appearance that is flawless as this appears unnatural. If you've got dark circles around your eyes, you can make them lighter by applying a light reflecting concealer which will make your face appear more radiant. your face. Apply a tiny amount of concealer to the corner of the eyes, and blend it outwards. After applying foundation and concealer, apply a tiny amount of translucent loose powder on the forehead and the nose with a clean brush to make the makeup last longer.

Eyes

The aim is to naturally draw attention to the eyes. It's a matter of personal preference, however I have noticed that a natural look of smokey eyes enhances the appearance of most faces and takes the attention from the face. Apply a base eyeshadow that's a similar shade to your skin on the lid , from the crease to the eyebrow using a smooth soft eyeshadow brush. Next, apply a darker shade (choose an eyeshadow that complements the colour of your eyes) If the eyes of your blue, go for orange, peach bronze, or gold. If you're green eyed, choose pink, purple hues, red shades as well as rose gold. If you're brown, opt for warm blue shades, for example, plum nude or green tones. If you have hazel eyes, opt for the warm tones of brown, gold green or purple. Use one of the colors using the same brush to the eye socket with gentle circular movements. gently sweep it under the eyes. Take a second shade and place it under the eye with a small blender brush. Sweep it to the outside of the eye. After that, blend upwards to the socket using the soft brush. Apply a generous coating of black mascara.

Lips

A lipstick shade which is a bit more vibrant than your natural color looks fantastic when paired with a natural smokey eyes and can brighten your face in general. An easy guide to selecting the right color - stay away from naked lipsticks since they can cause you to appear drab. When you're wearing cool tones (a red, pink, or blueish tone to your skin) pick the lipstick that has cool undertones (purple or blue with a cool undertone). When you're dealing with warm undertones (a golden, yellow or olive-tone to your skin) then go for warm shades such as coral, orange or reds that have the orange tone. For neutral tones (a mixture of yellow and pink) then the majority of shades are suitable for your skin. I suggest trying different shades to determine which ones can brighten your skin.

Application

Make sure your lips are prepared using a lip scrub and then followed by lip balm you can apply lip balm then gently massage your lips with a dry brush. Choose a lipliner pencil that matches your shade of lipstick. Apply gentle strokes of feathery line to define the lips' edges. Lips are filled in with an even coat of lipstick, then apply the lipstick on top, then blot it off, apply a second coat of lipstick, and apply another blot.

Cheeks

The aim is to brighten up your face with a little color. Apply a bronzer on your cheek bones using an easy blusher brush. Use a shade that is similar of lipstick selected (again play around with colors to determine which shade works best for you) Apply it on the apples of your cheeks using the blusher brush, using gentle circular motions.

Mindset

Keep this in mind as it comes to come to an end. This means you won't suffer from acne forever, it's simply a skin issue .... It's not your acne!

If you're in a positive mental attitude, it will assist you through this phase of your life. It will continue to assist you in tackling any challenges life may throw your way.

Your mind is the perception of you and others.

If you believe that having acne is ugly, and that it's the first thing people observe about you, it doesn't help and ultimately makes you feel uneasy about your appearance. If, however, you believe that you're a gorgeous and pleasant person with acne and that it doesn't define you and you'll instantly feel happier about yourself.

To be sure that your attitude is working for you and is not causing you to be unhappy, take note of all your thoughts and beliefs that you believe initially about yourself. For instance, I'm not confident I'm a failure I am a kind person, I love helping others etc.

Once you've recorded all your beliefs, both negative and positive, take an honest look and make changes to your beliefs that make you feel unhappy about your self.

Do the same with regard to the things you believe about others, for instance People are judgemental and rude, people have good intentions People are looking for the best of other people.

Once you've completed this you should now have two sets with positive belief systems that are working for you rather than against you. You'll be aware of negative beliefs that are hindering you.

Then think about how you would behave and behave if you were a believer in these new ideas, and then take action.

Focus your attention and thoughts on the positive aspects of your existence to ensure that you feel confident when you walk around with your head up and shoulders back, and with confidence!

One tip that can make you feel more confident when speaking to others is to concentrate on them , not you. take note of how they're experiencing and what you can accomplish to help make them feel better about themselves. Be sure to communicate clearly, with a smile and maintain eye contact.

Chapter 8: Acne Action Plan Putting It All Together

The Holistic Approach

As we have discussed in previous chapters , there are many aspects that can cause acne. Therefore, it is beneficial to adopt an overall treatment for acne.

You must ensure your digestion, your brain as well as your daily skincare routine.

Daily Rituals

You must have routines for your day to ensure you're taking good care of your areas every day.

I would suggest that you have an early morning routine so that you can get the majority of it completed early so that begin your day in a positive way.

Below is an illustration of my morning routine You can modify this to your own needs.

6.00 am - get up and write in my journal three things you are thankful for. This immediately boosts your mood. Drink a large glass of water that is warm that has the juice from a half lemon squeezed in it.

This will alkalize your body, calming your body down and ease any discomfort.

6.15 to am take an easy yoga class There are a lot of classes in yoga on YouTube and you can practice this from the convenience of your own home. This can help increase your strength and ease your mind and body.

7.00 - AM take a 10 minute meditation. and you will find many recorded meditations that are guided on YouTube. If you find the 10 minutes difficult, then start with five minutes. The practice will build your confidence and soothe your mind. It will it will also help to calm your entire body.

7.15 - AM: Do your routine for skincare and apply your makeup if you would like.

8.00 AM - go on for the rest of the day. Work, school, college etc.

Here's an example of how to incorporate the concepts discussed in your routine.

9.00 am - Take a class in the juice of celery. It can be made the night before and then taken to class in the bottle. You'll need a small handful of celery to make one large glass of juice from celery. Cleanse the celery and juice it with an juicer, or if you're making it ahead of the next day , then pour it in the glass bottle and put it in the refrigerator. If you don't own the juicer, then clean the celery, then chop it into pieces that are small and then place it in the blender along with 100ml of water filtered to blend. After that, strain the mix into a glass with an nut milk bag when you're preparing it for the following day, strain it into a glass and then empty into a bottle to keep in the refrigerator. The advantages that you get from drinking the juice of celery is that you're eating raw greens which are loaded with minerals and vitamins, it's an alkalizing drink for your body, and also helps boost the stomach acid in your body to improve digestion and improve your gut health.

10.30 am - Eat an easy breakfast. Oatmeal and blueberries are an excellent example.

11.00 am - consume any supplements you've taken, e.g probiotics, vitamins and probiotics.

1.00 pm - have nutritious lunch, such as tuna salad, soup made from scratch as well as chickpea salad.

3.00 pm - If you'd like to have a snack take a bite of fruit or a handful of almonds.

5.00 pm - once your work day is over, perform a mild aerobic exercise for 30 minutes, whether it's a walk in nature, a jog or an aerobic exercise from YouTube. Be sure not to exert yourself too much and you'd like your workout to be aerobic and not morph to anaerobic workout. When you go from anaerobic to aerobic exercise, it is a sign that you're exercising with no oxygen and this will put too much stress to your body. It is easy to tell if you are doing aerobic exercises when you are unable to talk as you're exhausted. Aerobic exercise can boost overall health and well-being, as well being good for your mental wellbeing.

6.30 pm - Eat your healthy meal, excellent examples include salmon and vegetables and brown rice as well as vegetable and chicken. Always include some vegetables that are green into your meals.

Make sure you're drinking plenty of water throughout the day.

10.00 pm - complete your evening routine of skincare. Include your additional skincare routine 2-3 times per week, such as exfoliation and mask.

As mentioned previously, it is vital to get a good night's sleep to help balance your hormones. Here are 3 strategies for getting a good night's rest.

1.) Do not use your device or smartphone for an hour prior to when you go to go to bed. The blue light that is emitted by your tablet and phone blocks the hormone melatonin that is the hormone responsible for making you sleepy.

2.) Place your smartphone and tablet in airplane mode prior to going to bed if you are sleeping close to them. When WiFi is turned on, it emits electromagnetic fields that can hinder the production of Melatonin.

3.) Light from the sun or artificial sources will also inhibit Melatonin production. Therefore, ensure you have a bedroom that is dark prior to going to bed.

Chapter 9: My Experiment With Acne Acne

As with many who suffer from acne, I started to break out during my teenage years. At the age of middle school, around thirteen, I noticed pimples popping up all over my face. At first, I would see a couple of pimples on my face here and there. As I began my first year of high school my skin was in the worst shape and would stay the same for two years. Being a victim of this anxiety during such a vulnerable period during my lifetime was a challenge. A majority of my friends were clear-skinny, and they didn't understand my issues and concerns. I wasn't confident with makeup and put on foundation and concealer in an attempt to hide my face. I didn't realize that the products I put on my face was causing problems for my delicate skin as well as making acne more aggravated.

To top it off the prescriptions I received from my dermatologist (such as tretinoin, retin-a benzoyl peroxide, clindamycin and benzoyl) affected my skin to the point of irritation. Every product I bought at the pharmacy contained ingredients that I couldn't pronounce. The chemicals contained in these product caused my face to dry and itch, burn and peel.

To make matters worse my diet was a disaster. Restaurant food and fast food made up the majority portions of meals. The old saying that says... it's true that you truly are what you consume. The oily foods were shining through. The skin of my was oily as well as streaky.

Discoveries of Natural Skin Care

Another few years went through as my battle with acne grew. This was when I began taking care of my skin in my own control. My dermatologist and the pharmacy provided me with the results I required. Now, I'm 20 years old, and my acne is clearing over the past year following a series of efforts. Now , I realize that the chemicals I put to my face are just short-term remedies. They helped to treat the problem externally, however every single one of the processes and bacteria inside that part of my body was ignored. The solution was found to be to address my acne from its source (the within my own body).

After absorbing all these facts, I came to the conclusion that, in order to improve my appearance on the outside it is essential to take treatment of my entire body and not solely my face. This brought me to the idea of natural skin treatment. My concept about natural care of the skin is comprised of a variety of elements such as natural skin care products that are applied to the skin and diet, exercising being stress-free and living a more healthy and mindful life.

Chapter 10: Essential Oils For Natural Skin Care

The use of essential oils is among my most preferred (and most efficient) ways to treat acne. Essential oils come from plants, which is done by distilling them using the help of steam as well as water. The result is concentrated oils which can be applied on the skin or diffused for aromatherapy to improve the health for your health. They have antibacterial properties that naturally combat acne-causing bacteria. If applied topically or eaten the nutrients are absorbed by the body, and offer antioxidants that fight the damage to skin cells.

Prior to applying essential oils to your skin, it's crucial to perform an experiment with a patch. Place a tiny amount of the oil on a small area of your skin to determine whether it reacts negatively or results in an eruption. Essential oils are extremely concentrated and certain skin types may be extremely sensitive to their power.

Here's a list of my top essential oils I apply to your skin, and their advantages:

Essential oil of Tea Tree My go-to oil. This oil has given me the most efficient and noticeable effects for the acne I suffer from. Tea tree oil has antimicrobial (fights diseases and the bad bacteria you shouldn't have within the body) properties as well as anti-inflammatory properties that can reduce their size as well as dry the pimples out. It also breaks down the dirt and oil that is stuck in your pores, reducing the appearance of acne. By inhaling the oil and diffusing it, the benefits to your whole body. Tea tree oil is absorbed by into the respiratory tract, it ultimately is absorbed into the bloodstream, helping to cleanse your body of bacteria that cause acne.

To apply tea tree oils on the skin, I would recommend using tea tree oil for an application for spot treatments because it is extremely strong and concentrated. Use three drops onto the cotton ball, then dab it on the area of your concern.

Don't be worried in the event that you experience the sensation of burning, this is normal. Tea tree oil is killing the bacteria on your skin. But, take care not to get caught up and apply the pure oil of tea trees on your face. I have learned this lesson the hard way! Too much use could cause your skin to become irritated and itchy.

If you'd like to apply it on your entire face, it is possible to dilute it first with water before applying it to more areas. I recommend 1 cup of water to every 3 to 4 drops oil when applied in large amounts to treat acne.

How to diffuse tea tree oil several ways of diffusing tea tree oils get the most benefits it offers for your skin.

Simply place a few drops of oil on an item of cloth and place it close to you. It will then move across the air close to your body for inhalation.

Utilize a diffuser. That's what that I use the most. The diffuser can be described as a device that mixes oil and water inside the machine. It produces steam that can be absorbed by the whole room. The steam that you inhale releases oils into blood vessels and circulates through your entire body. This is a wonderful method to take in the scent of the oil in your home and to help create healthy air quality in your workplace or living space.

The stove should be filled to the top: Pour a pan with water in part and add between five and 6 drops of tea tree oils. Make sure the heat is high enough that the container steams but it does not boil. This method functions in the similar way to diffusers and diffuses the air with this therapeutic oil.

Lavender Essential Oil - This oil performs in the same ways like tea tree oil. It's antimicrobial and supplies the body with antioxidants. In addition lavender oil can be used to heal dry, acne-damaged skin and diminish the appearance of scars and spots. Lavender oil is known for its relaxing scent which promotes relaxation, sleep and stress-reliefand all of these contribute to healthy and radiant skin.

For lavender oil use on your skin: Place the oil in small amounts onto a ball of cotton, then apply it directly to the skin area you wish to treat. It can also be applied to your temples or wrists to allow it to pass into your skin and to reap the benefits.

to diffuse the lavender essential oil Lavender oil can be used to diffuse in a variety of ways that tea tree oil is. But there are alternatives to experiment benefit from this oil that is a miracle to help your skin.

Your pillow In the middle of your pillow case, put some drops on your pillow and place it on your head. As you lie down on your bed, the fragrance will give you a sense of peace and help with stress relief.

The bath Pour a little water into your bath with water and add couple of drops of lavender. The bath water helps diffuse the scent and allows it to soak in your skin while you soak in the warm bath.

Essential oils are the best method you can treat the skin way it was intended to look. They don't contain harmful chemicals, preservatives or harsh chemicals and contain no ingredients that cannot be recognized. It's an easy method to make sure that your skin isn't getting any substances that can cause irritation to your body and trigger breakouts of acne. Simply good old-fashioned plant love and take care of your skin. Lavender oil is a great method to lessen stress and treat your acne. In the next section, I'll provide a brief explanation about how to reduce acne-causing stress through exercising!

Chapter 11: How To Treat Acne Through Exercise And Stress Reduction

As we know, the brain is home to a variety of nerves that are linked to the body. That means when you're stressed out the body is also feeling the results.

Your skin constantly produces sebum, an oily compound This oil is designed to maintain your skin's suppleness. The causes of acne are stress, since the cells within the body which produce sebum possess receptors that are able to recognize stress hormones. The body produces more sebum when you're stressed. The sebum production that is excessive blends with dead skin cells shed from your skin and results in blocked pores. This results in breakouts from acne.

Exercise is an excellent instrument to treat acne since it produces endorphins that boost moods in your body. Additionally, it gets your blood flowing , which increases circulation, and also to supply oxygen to the cells of your skin. Oxygen helps your skin eliminate acne-causing waste.

Methods to cleanse your body of stress

Hiking: The benefits of hiking go beyond just running on a treadmill. The outdoors can provide your body with sun and fresh air. It also provides the tranquil music of nature. These all work well in calming your body and refocusing your mind. When you hike, you are able to use a wider variety of muscles due to changing trails as well as the climbs uphill. This means you're getting more energy and generating an increase in blood flow to heal your acne. Find a scenic trail near you and start getting your heart beating!

Yoga: Yoga is the practice of stretching your body while control of your breathing. Both of these can bring relaxation to your tight limbs as well as to your racing thoughts. Yoga can aid in healing acne as the stretching increases blood flow and elimination. The wide variety of yoga poses will induce deep breathing and provide lots of oxygen into your face.

My Top Yoga Poses for Treating Acne

Shoulder Stand- This particular posture assists to treat your skin by improving circulation. By elevating your legs above your head, they increase the flow of blood to your face. Here's how to accomplish it:

Begin by lying on your back flat with your hands placed by your sides.

Once you're ready to lift your legs, place your feet on the ceiling, one at one at a time. Put your hands in your lower back for assistance. Make sure that your body's weight is on your shoulders and not on your neck. This could result in injuries and pain.

Make sure your elbows are flat on the ground to support you.

Be sure your thighs are connected

Do this for 30 seconds

Slowly lower your legs one at a time , until you're back in your the original position.

Cobra Pose-Cobra poses help cleanse your skin in several ways. The primary reason is that doing this pose awakens your facial muscles. This stimulates your skin cells to regenerate their own. The deep stretch also stimulates the abdominal organs region; a healthy stomach results in healthier skin.

Here's how to accomplish it:

Begin by lying flat on your stomach, with the feet's tops looking down.

Put your hands under your shoulders. Your fingers should point directly toward the direction of your face.

Your elbows should be tucked into the sides of your body.

By pressing your body against the heels of your feet as well as your pubic bone raise your chest off the floor gradually. Your back should be able to feel stretched and not strained.

For a deeper stretch, extend your shoulders backwards, then press your chest forward.

Straighten your arms to increase the stretch in your back.

Turn your head slightly back and look up towards the ceiling. Do this for 30 seconds or until you are ready to take a break.

Begin by lowering your body to the floor as you exhale.

Remember that performing these exercises or going on hikes for a day won't help your acne. It is essential to adhere to a schedule and perform them regularly to manage the stress you experience to enable your body to feel the benefits of stress reduction.

Controlled Breathing to Lower Stress

Alongside stretching and physical exercise is breathing. These exercises will let your lungs breathe easier and boost the amount of oxygen you get Be conscious that you breathe is vital to ensure a healthy flow of blood.

How can breathing be affected by Stress?

If you are feeling stressed and discomfort, it is possible to can end breath too quickly. The result is that excessive oxygen into the bloodstream and alters the balance between carbon dioxide and oxygen. The result is a throw off balance of pH, which can cause anxiety, stress and irritation. These feelings can trigger breakouts of acne due to the fact that, as I stated at the beginning of this article skin cells contain receptors for stress hormones.

How to Control Your Breathing and Relax your Body

A method of breathing I've been using for the past two years has not been able to meet my expectations. It's a method that I learned in yoga classes named "Ujjayi." Ujjayi breathing is based on breathing through the nose, creating an sound that is like the sound of the ocean. My yoga instructor informed me that this style of breathing can help regulate blood pressure, which can reduce stress in your body.

How to Train Ujjayi Breathing

Take a deep breath and locate a comfortable place to sit. I like to sit criss-cross.

Make sure you seal your lips, then take an DEEP inhale with your nose. The inhale last for about 6 seconds.

Take a deep breath for 3 seconds.

Inhale through your nostrils, allowing your exhale to last for about 6 minutes or so until you are completely empty.

Repeat the exercise as many times as you need or want until your head is calm as well as your body in a calm state.

The most amazing thing about this method to ease your mind is that it can use it wherever you want. This breathing method is always able to help me relax. I use Ujjayi when I'm upset, anxious, or stressed and it immediately calms my body.

Chapter 12: Dietary Tips For Healthful Skin

In my experience, my diet does affect my skin. If I consume refined and sugary food I notice a change in the appearance of my skin and the feel.

Junk food is made up of many artificial chemicals that can lead to an accumulation of toxins within your body. If your body is stuffed overflowing with toxic substances your liver (which is the organ that processes your body's toxins, and then filters them out) becomes overwhelmed and is unable to rid your body of toxins fast enough. Your body then has extra toxins it needs to come up with other ways to eliminate; and in some cases, it will do this through the pores of your skin. This can cause pimples.

How I Changed My diet to fight Acne

The process of readjusting my diet wasn't as difficult as I had hoped it was going to be. Don't be intimidated by this aspect, it's far simpler than you imagine. The most important aspect of diet is to ensure that your body is getting everything it requires to perform. Your skin will be thankful for it! Here are some of the key modifications I made that have brought me visible outcomes:

I began eating organic food whenever I could. Organic vegetables and fruits are produced without pesticides or GMOs (genetically engineered organisms intended to make the food grow more quickly more attractive, look better and protect against bugs). Organic meat and eggs are produced with no use of growth hormones , and the animals that make the food are fed organic grains and grass. Growth hormones are administered to animals to accelerate their growth (cows produce more meat that can be sold) as well as the amount of products they create (hormones are used to help chickens create larger eggs). Organic food choices ensure that you are keeping those undesirable chemicals and hormones out of your body. Take this this way: If you eat products or animals that is treated with artificial antibiotics or hormones, certain chemicals are likely to enter your body.

The toxic chemicals and hormones could alter your body's hormones, causing breakouts of acne.

I limit my meat intake. As I stated in the previous paragraph, eating food that is treated with hormones may affect your hormones. The hormonal imbalance can cause acne.

I steer clear of processed foods rich in sugar. As I've mentioned previously processed foods aren't healthy for the body. They release toxins from the ingredients which can cause breakouts of acne.

To sum everything down, just look for the most natural food you can get. Make sure to stay clear of any the use of additives in your food, and make sure you read the labels to know precisely what's in your body. Make sure you are buying foods with natural or organic GMO labeling. It is also important to supply your skin with antioxidants and vitamins to maintain its health.

Foods to nourish your skin

To heal your skin and improve your general health, eat foods that contain these ingredients:

Lots of antioxidants-Foods that contain vitamin A, C, and E are among the most vital in your diet. These antioxidants are designed to shield the skin cells from being damaged by sun radiation and also provide you with a radiant glow. Beta carotene is also part of the antioxidant class and converts into vitamin A inside the body.

Vitamin A: Onions carrots and squash. Also spinach bell peppers, sweet potatoes and goat cheese

Vitamin C: Oranges (or juice), broccoli, tomatoes, pineapple, brussels sprouts

Vitamin E Avocado Olive oil canola oil, almonds hazelnuts and asparagus

Omega-3 fatty acids - Omega-3s help reduce inflammation (which could heal pimples) within your body. Furthermore they assist in controlling your mood and the hormones that keep your breakouts in check. A few examples of foods that are rich in omega-3s are:

Salmon, sardines, mackerel, trout, tuna, shrimp

Eggs butter, eggs, milk and yogurt

Walnuts and soybeans (cooked) navy beans, walnuts

Cauliflower, kale (cooked), blackberries, pomegranates

My experience has been that the addition of these nutrients and vitamins into my diet has helped in the healing of my skin. A further noticeable change in my face is the fact that it appears healthier, more moisturized and doesn't scar as easily due to acne breakouts.

Chapter 13: Lifestyle Improvements To Better Skin Health

Based on the information you've gathered in this book taking care of your skin needs care in every aspect of your daily life. Your habits through your daily routine can affect the appearance and the feel that your face has. This chapter will tell you about the bad habits that I discovered that had negative effects to my complexion. Here are some tips that you can follow to treat acne-prone skin:

Make sure you remove your makeup prior to going to bed. This is the most crucial method of ensuring the health of your skin. Your makeup accumulates dirt throughout the day, which could cause damage to the skin. While you're sleeping your body rests and recuperating itself. Doing your makeup in the late at night isn't allowing the skin breathe or heal from the pressure it experienced throughout the day. Also the act of putting your makeup on during are asleep can cause pores to become clogged and can lead to acne breakouts.

Change your pillowcase each week. Think about the amount of bacteria and dirt that your face and hair accumulate throughout the day. Then suppose you are going to bed and do not wash either. A soiled pillow is what you'll end with. It's simple to ignore. At the point you go to mattress at night, after your day, you're unlikely to do anything other than lie down. It is beneficial for the cleanliness and glow of your skin to wash your pillowcase every week at least. This will ensure that you're lying your face on a clean surface so that it can relax and replenish.

Drink more water - As you're aware, the human body is made up largely of water. It is crucial for water to flow through your body to flush out the toxins and bacteria. If you're not water-hydrated, your body's wastes could accumulate and increase the likelihood of developing breakouts.

Make sure to wash your makeup brushes. This is the same principle like cleaning your pillowcases. Bacteria build up on your makeup brushes whenever you use them. You can leave them out on the counter in

your bathroom, or even share them with your acquaintances. It is crucial to wash all makeup tools (I wash them after two or three times) to get rid of the pore-clogging bacteria which can cause acne breakouts.
The habits you adopt along with what you've learned from this book will surely put you on the road to better skin.

Chapter 14: A Home Remedies For Acne Recipes

There are many substances that come from nature that could help your skin, so why not make use of these? Finding different methods of taking care of your skin is among the most exciting aspects of this. In this section I'll discuss some of the recipes I have used to combat my acne. In addition, you will learn about the advantages of these ingredients that are natural many of which are at home!

Turmeric Acne Cream

Ingredients:

1 teaspoon of turmeric powder

1/2 tsp lemon juice

Coconut oil (desired quantity)

Instructions:

Mix the turmeric powder and lemon juice in a medium-sized bowl

Pour coconut oil into the mixture as you stir the mixture until it becomes a smooth paste

Apply the paste on your face, then take it off after it has dried completely.

The coconut oil, the lemon juice and turmeric are three of the most potent natural ingredients for treating acne you can locate! The turmeric powder is a great way to exfoliate your skin while lemon juice helps unclog your pores and kills the bad bacteria that cause breakouts. The coconut oil assists in taking away excess oils from your skin while helping to keep your skin moisturized and preventing dryness. Make sure to use this paste not more than once a week because lemon juice may affect the pH levels of your facial oils. Additionally, exfoliating should be performed no more than two times per week. This is due to the fact that excessive exfoliation may cause inflammation of skin cells.

Acne Fighting Lavender Recipe
Ingredients:
12 OZ bottle of witch-hazel
7 drops of lavender oil
1 teaspoon apple cider vinegar
Instructions:
Simply mix all ingredients together

Apply the mix on the areas of your face that are prone to acne using a cotton swab cotton ball

Lavender oil and apple cider vinegar and witch hazel have been acknowledged to be effective in naturally reducing acne breakouts. Apple cider vinegar has antibacterial properties and witch hazel can help repair skin cells and decrease inflammation. The three ingredients also help prevent future breakouts of acne when they are used frequently.

The Honey-Almond Exfoliating Scrub (ingredients that are listed for various uses)

Ingredients

Four teaspoons honey

One teaspoon extra virgin olive oil (EVOO)

5 tablespoons of almonds crushed

Instructions:

Combine your honey with EVOO, honey and almonds that have been crushed in the blender

Let the mixture sit for 24 hours.

Use the cleanser directly on your face, applying gentle pressure. It will target the areas that are prone to acne.

Make a scrub every 3-5 days to prevent and relieve acne breakouts on your own.

Honey helps help keep your skin moisturized and reduce irritation. Olive oil that is extra virgin supplies the skin with Vitamin E as well as regenerating the skin's tissues. Additionally almonds are also rich in vitamin E, and they can aid in healing acne and preventing the appearance of scars.

Papaya Face Mask

Ingredients

1 fresh papaya

Instructions

Start by washing your face.

Peel the papaya

Mash your fruit's flesh (this can be done with the blender or with a hand). Make sure it's soft but not too thick to adhere to the skin.

Place the mask on for 15 minutes

Cleanse the mask with the water that is lukewarm.

Papaya fruit is extremely rich in vitamin A, which acts as an anti-oxidant for skin. It also aids in the elimination decomposing skin cells which helps in cleansing your pores and helping to prevent breakouts.

The masks also assist in healing any acne marks. Next chapter is going to tell you in more detail on how to treat acne scars and marks.

Chapter 15: What To Restore Acne Marks And Scars

Now, you've managed to get the acne out of your system and started the process of healing. But what happens to those lingering acne scars that will not disappear?

In the beginning There is a distinction in acne scars and scars. Acne marks appear flat on your skin however, they appear to be more dark (red and purple) than the other skin tones. The reason for this is that your skin produces a lot of melanin (pigment on your skin) as it tries to recover after the acne. Acne scars appear as indentures on your skin result of your skin seeking to repair itself after an acne breakout. When your skin attempts to heal the scar by generating new tissue to cover the mark but sometimes it fails to create enough tissue to fill in the indentation which leads to craters.

Acne marks typically fade by themselves or after treatment. In the case of acne scars that are indented, they are more difficult to treat and usually require more intensive treatment, such as laser treatments. But, the solutions I'll demonstrate will still be beneficial to your acne scars with nutrients and restore your appearance.

Removing Acne Scars using Rosehip Oil

It was (and remains) my life-saving oil! The oil was the cherry in my quest to heal my skin. I had lots of acne scars that remained as well as an uneven complexion. Rosehip oil helped smooth my skin and erase my purple and red acne marks. Additionally it also helped reduce the size of my pores that I have on my skin.

Warn

Don't think of rosehip oil as rose oil. The rose oil is derived from the rose petals and therefore contains many fragrances. The scent can be a irritation to the skin and may aggravate your acne. Remember that prior to applying any oil to your skin, it's crucial to perform an experiment with a patch. Apply the oil to only a tiny area of your skin to make sure that it won't cause an itch. Some types of skin may be affected by these natural oils.

The oil of rosehip comes by the seed of wild rosebushes. It's a rich source in vitamin A and vitamin C that are potent antioxidants that help to rejuvenate your skin cells and even out the coloration of your skin. This oil is among the most effective remedies for acne scars with indentation. It aids in rebuilding collagen within your skin, that can help make the scars less visible.

How do you use Rosehip Oil to Treat your Marks

I have had great results the use of rosehip oil for an oil to moisturize my skin. Rosehip oil, however, can be utilized in numerous ways to treat your skin.

For a moisturizing effect, wash your face, then pat your skin dry. Apply the rosehip oils of two drops onto your fingertips and rub it onto your neck and face. Two drops is enough. Keep in mind that a small amount goes far.

Mix it in with your face moisturizer. Place the your desired amount of moisturizer in your hands. Add 2 to 3 drops of the rosehip oil to your moisturizer. Mix the two together with your hands. After that, apply the moisturizer to your the face like you would normally.

Mix it with essential lavender oil. Combine the moisturizing qualities of lavender oil with the healing properties of rosehip oil to treat your scars. Combine two drops each of the oils and apply it to your face prior to bed.

Tips Regarding Rosehip Oil

It is recommended to buy rosehip oil that has been cold-pressed. This signifies that the extraction procedure didn't involve heating and therefore, it is able to retain the healing properties of rosehip oil.

Be sure to keep the rosehip oil in a cool, dark, and cool space. It's easy to go bad in the event of exposure to extreme temperatures.

Treatment of Acne marks with Apple Cider Vinegar and Honey

Honey and ACV contain anti-inflammatory and antibacterial properties. Both of them will help prevent the growth of acne-causing bacteria while also calming your skin while removing the acne-causing marks.

How to use ACV and Honey on your skin

You'll require:

2 tablespoons honey

One tablespoon of ACV.

Water

For use on your skin:

Mix ACV and honey in a bowl

Mix with water and add water.

With a cotton ball apply the mix on the areas affected

Rinse off after 15 minutes.

Use Lemon to Remove Acne Marks and Scars

Lemons are rich of vitamin C. Vitamin C helps with the creation of collagen within your skin. This assists your skin in renewing itself and fill in the acne-related wrinkles. It also reduces the skin's redness. Lemon helps fade those acne marks that are red due to its exfoliating properties. This means that it can remove the layers of skin that are causing the redness and diminish the marks.

How to use Lemon for your skin

Begin by cutting the lemon in half before squeeze the juice into the bowl

A cotton ball should be dipped in the juice, then apply it to the marks you have made

Allow it to sit for a few minutes. Make sure you rinse it off in case it begins feeling hot or uncomfortable.

Tips for Using Lemon on your skin

Lemon juice can trigger the skin's production of melanin (the pigment that your skin produces). If you have dark skin, I don't suggest applying lemon juice to your skin since it may create darker spots.

Lemon may cause irritation to certain people's skin. Be sure to conduct the test with a patch first.

Chapter 16: Everything About Acne

You glance in the mirror and then you notice something that wasn't there before. There's the appearance of acne on your face!

Be assured that getting acne doesn't mean that you're done with the world. It is easy to find an array of acne treatments you can use to get rid of that acne across your skin. The battle between you and your acne will never be simple however, it's one that you will be victorious.

Do not enter battle without the proper ammunition. Know your opponent.

Is acne a condition?

Acne: A definition

Acne (medical name: Acne vulgaris) is an infection of the skin that affects the oil glands located in the hair follicles' bases.

Acne usually occurs at puberty time, since it is the time when the oil glands in your body, also known as sebaceous glands, begin to come into life because of the adrenal glands producing hormones. Acne typically appears during puberty, but for some, it can last throughout life.

Acne doesn't develop overnight. It's an ongoing process that can last for several weeks prior to the appearance of that blemish. It's a good thing that you can keep your acne at bay or use treatments and/or treatments to take the pimples away from your skin.

What causes Acne?

Your skin is the most important organ in your body. It is responsible for a variety of tasks, like fighting off illnesses and controlling your temperature. If you take care to treat it correctly, you'll face no skin issues However, there will be times that you'll be experiencing acne.

Acne usually occurs at the time of puberty and more specifically, during the teenage years. The hormone levels, specifically testosterone levels, increase in this time.

Oil is released naturally through your pores, so that your skin is protected and dry. However, since there's an increase of hormones, you will see an increase in the production of oil from the glands of your skin.

What is the time when acne occurs? Acne is caused when oil mixes in dead skin cells, and ends in clogging your pores. Bacteria may then grow in this mix. Once this mixture is absorbed in tissues, you'll notice swelling, pus, and redness. So there you go You've are suffering from red bumps that are sometimes referred to as pimples.

Utilizing medicines such as corticosteroids and lithium may cause acne. If you're worried about this, you should talk to your physician about it.

Who can get Acne?

Are you suffering from acne? It's not just you. And it's not only teens who suffer from it. Acne is among the most frequent skin issues. Have you ever heard that infants are also susceptible to acne? The reason is that hormones are transmitted to the babies by their mothers. If a baby is stressed during birth, his body releases hormones that may cause acne. Young children and adults may also suffer from acne. That means that everybody can experience acne at some time in their lives.

Acne The Symptoms

Acne isn't confined to pimples by itself. Acne sufferers may have any of these:

* Whiteheads
* Blackheads
* Cysts
* Papules.
* Nodules
* Pustules (what is commonly referred to as 'pimples').

Acne is not only visible on the face, but on the chest, neck as well as the back, shoulders, neck and various other areas of the body.

Affects of Acne

Acne isn't as dangerous in the way it is, however it is painful, especially when it gets extreme. It can, however, cause emotional stress.

If you've experienced acne at some point in your lifetime, you're aware of the negative effects of acne that extend beyond the the skin. It's important to safeguard yourself to avoid the negative effects that it can cause.

Why would you want to avoid acne? Because having acne can result in:

Dark Spots

You've waited for years to see the day that your acne will heal and disappear for good. But , like a terrible broken-hearted relationship, those dark patches will remain in your mind and bring back the your acne caused.

Since the acne healed, they'll eventually disappear and be disappear. Of course, you'd prefer to not suffer from acne at all in the first place, to avoid dark spots since it can take several months or even years for them to fade.

Permanent Scars

People who suffer from acne cysts or nodules usually have scars when the acne is gone. However, there is a chance that you can prevent getting these marks if you're still a young person (around 8-12 years older) and that you have your skin examined by a dermatologist earlier.

Acne-related history in your family ought to be an incentive to visit a dermatologist when you experience acne, so that you can get the proper treatment right away, which will reduce the chances of acquiring the appearance of scars.

Self-esteem is low.

It is common for people to feel uneasy when they suffer from acne. They feel unworthy and insecure and don't desire to go out to socialize with loved ones and friends. Many even decide to skip classes or work. This can greatly impact their performance, and absences can cause more issues - and this is not just due to acne.

It's true that acne can be thought of as the most widespread skin problem however, it can still impact the emotions of those with acne. It could make you feel lonely and less attractive.

Depression

Certain people have the self-esteem issue; others result in depression. This can cause many negative impacts on a person, and may even cause suicide in some people.

What is the severity? Teens, in particular tend to think their faces are ugly due to acne and then end in harming themselves due to it.

It's not necessary to go this far. Be careful not to cause harm to yourself by having acne. There are a variety of treatment options you can try. There's always some hope.

Natural Acne Treatments

There is no need to immediately use medications or operations to combat acne. Acne is now treated with natural remedies like household products as well as essential oils.

Home Treatments

The good news is that it's true!

There is no need to travel for a long distance to treat your acne. There are plenty of common items you can utilize to combat acne, and also reduce the chance of getting scars around your skin.

Take a look at these household items and discover how they combat acne.

Apple Cider Vinegar

You've likely heard about the benefits that apple cider vinegar has to offer. It's also popular as a treatment for acne. How?

Apple cider vinegar is a source of the acid lactic that can help reduce the inflammation and swelling caused by acne. It also aids in the dissolution of old skin cells and kills bacteria and cleanse dirt, makeup, oil and dirt that has accumulated on the skin.

Vinegar is also an antiseptic. You could make use of the vinegar to make a cleanser for your skin, helping to remove blemishes fast. It also helps to restore the pH levels of the skin.

How can you make use of apple cider vinegar to treat acne? Two methods:

* Mix apple cider vinegar using water. A portion of cider apple and 2 parts of water might work, but you could consider adding more water if you suffer from sensitive skin.

* You may also take apple cider vinegar by mixing the vinegar and water, and then drinking the mix once per day.

It is important to be patient when making use of apple cider vinegar however, since the effects can not be felt immediately. The time frame for results varies depending on the individual. Some require waiting for weeks or days.

Make sure to apply sunscreen if the skin treated is going exposure to direct sunlight. Not using sunscreen could cause sunburn.

Baking soda

Baking soda, also known as sodium bicarbonate is also a chemical that is utilized in treating acne. It's not hard to locate baking soda, or perhaps find it in your pantry.

What is the reason baking soda is the most popular method for treating acne? It's because it helps remove the excess oil as well as dry up pimples. It aids in fixing the skin's pH imbalance , which can cause the development of acne. It also has anti-inflammatory and mild antiseptic properties that help reduce the inflammation caused by acne.

What is the best way to use baking soda for acne treatment?

A good way to do this is by mixing baking soda and water. Apply the paste to the skin once a week. Another option is to add 2-3 grams of the paste into your favorite shampoo to lessen the appearance of the appearance of acne on the hairline. Apart from that additional options, you can add 100g baking soda to your bath water . Not only will your skin feel rejuvenated, but it will also be protected from breakouts.

Be aware when baking soda as it could cause stinging or burning. Make a skin patch or try it before applying it. It is safe to use regularly but be cautious when you have skin that is sensitive.

Honey

If there's a different item that has multiple uses, that you can utilize for acne and acne, it's honey. It has anti-inflammatory, healing, and antibacterial properties reduce the chances of an breakouts.

Honey has been a great cosmetic treatment for a variety of skin problems These concerns include acne. Its osmotic effects absorb water and produces hydrogen peroxide. This clears acne and kills the bacteria. It releases essential oils that help it act as an ointment.

Honey is a great ingredient to treat acne?

Honey can be sprayed to the skin for masks, and put aside for 20-30 minutes. Cleanse your face afterward and make sure not to leave any marks. Make sure to do this at least every two weeks.

It is also possible to mix oatmeal and honey into a paste to be applied to the face, and then left to dry for approximately 10 to 15 minutes. The face needs to be cleaned afterward and dried using the towel.

If you'd like to apply honey as is, just apply honey straight on the acne. You can also apply the bandage made of plastic (i.e. bands-aid) for covering the area and keep from creating an mess. The honey must be removed by soaking in water. Continue this each at night, until your acne is eliminated completely.

Be sure to cleanse your face, and get rid of all honey residue from your skin. This will leave you with clear, clear skin.

Ice

It is more of a short-term treatment rather than a long-term solution. Ice's coldness will assist in the reduction of redness and swelling.

What is the best way to use Ice to reduce acne?

It is possible to grab an ice cube, and then press directly onto the pimple which is swelling. wait for a few minutes for the pimple to take in the freezing cold of the ice.

Do not put the ice excessively long over your face, you'll get freezer burns if you do this.

Essential Oils

In addition to household items You can also search for essential oils that treat acne. They are a great source of help in the removal of the unsightly acne that appears visible on your face. They also help to moisturize your skin and improve the appearance of your skin and younger.

What kind of essential oils are you able to utilize?

Tea Tree Oil

It is among the most recommended essential oils for acne due to its antibacterial, anti-fungal , and anti-inflammatory properties. It's superior to other acne treatments as it protects against further damage and does not strip your skin the natural oil it produces.

How can you make use of Tea tree oils?

Put a few drops of the oil onto the cotton pad. Dab the oil on pimples and other spots that are affected. After a few hours the swelling and redness will lessen.

Rosemary

What makes rosemary a great option for acne treatment?

The oil of rosemary has antioxidant and anti-inflammatory properties. They can protect your skin from breakouts and irritations that acne can trigger. It's also not a comedogenic.

How can you apply rosemary to acne?

It is possible to use rosemary in the form of dropping small amounts oil on cotton swabs, then apply the oil to the skin. If you feel that you are stinging upon applying it, you can mix it with carrier oils, such as Jojoba oil and massage it onto the face.

Lemon

Lemons have a variety of purposes, and one of them is to create oils that can combat acne. It functions as an antiseptic, and it peels facial skin with natural. It aids in clearing acne and helps balance sebaceous glands, and balances sebaceous.

What is the best way to use lemon to treat acne?

A cotton ball place a few drops lemon oil. Apply it directly onto the affected and dry skin. It is important that you don't apply lemon oil to skin that will be exposed to direct sunlight. Wait for at least 72 hours to avoid irritation.

Lavender

What is the reason lavender is good for acne?

Lavender is an excellent acne treatment due to its ability to heal the skin. It can also help calm the skin and get rid of pimples.

How can you apply lavender for acne?

It is best to dilute essential oils prior to applying. Mix it into carrier oils like almond or olive oil. Apply the oil directly onto the skin using cotton swabs.

Oregano

Oregano is a different ideal acne treatment due to it's antiviral and antiseptic, and antibacterial properties. In addition, it reduces acne-causing bacteria and decreases redness and swelling.

How to Utilize:

Mix some drops of oregano oil into an ounce of water. Apply the solution directly on the acne with cotton balls, and allow it to go to dry over the face naturally.

What Food Affects Acne

It's now possible to tell that chocolate isn't the cause of acne. Pizza isn't the same. It is now time to celebrate.

You are the food you consume. The food you consume affects the body, particularly your skin. Food choices you make can cause or prevent acne. Which one will you pick?

Start by determining what foods can help you fight the battle against acne.

Prevention of Acne

Broccoli

Numerous studies have proven the health benefits of broccoli to the body. It's regarded as a "superfood that parents across the globe would like their children to consume. In addition to the other issues that broccoli can help to alleviate broccoli can also help get free of acne.

Broccoli is beneficial for skin health because it's high in Vitamin C. What's the reason we are we so fond of Vitamin C? It's because it works as an antioxidant. It reduces cortisol's stress hormone and assists in the production of collagen. In addition, broccoli is high in Vitamin E which is an antioxidant that can help keep pores from becoming blocked and magnesium.

Broccoli is also a great way to reduce inflammation thanks to the ingredient known as sulforaphane . It prevents your pimples from expanding and turning red.

Green Tea

Do you want to reduce acne? Consider green tea. Apart from treating ailments like headache, anxiety as well as depression, this may be used to treat other ailments as well.

What is the best way to use green tea to be used to treat acne?

Green tea can help reduce acne by reducing inflammation of the skin which reduces acne scars and rashes. It also aids in fighting acne-causing bacteria as well as lower the blood sugar level. Green tea drinking can result in less oil production.

It's not an 'all-purpose drink' which will totally eliminate the appearance of acne, particularly when your diet is a source of foods that cause acne However, what it can help with is to minimize the damage that could occur.

Don't let this stop you from enjoying green tea as it will improve your skin and improve overall health.

Brown Rice

Vitamin B as well as protein, magnesium, and a variety of antioxidants from brown rice. The consumption of brown rice can aid in reducing stress, which can lead to managing hormone levels and reducing breakouts.

Brown rice is a great source of food fiber and has a the lowest glycemic load, therefore, your body will digest it much more slowly. Also, it is a rich source of selenium which helps to keep the skin elastic and reduces inflammation.

Walnuts

In addition to preventing zombies from entering the well-known game Walnuts also help to stop acne from appearing on your face.

Walnuts are a rich source of essential fatty acids which provide the skin with numerous health benefits. Walnuts are a great option for people with dry skin as and for people suffering from eczema.

Walnuts are also high in Omega-3 fatty acids, which help to reduce the appearance of acne and reduce inflammation. under the control. A teaspoon of walnuts will enhance the Omega-3 fatty acids' power.

Avocado

Many may advise against eating avocados because of its fat content, however it's actually quite healthy to your complexion.

Avocado is loaded with nutrients like Vitamin C as well as Vitamin E; Vitamin C helps reduce skin inflammation and acts as a moisturizer for the skin. Vitamin E is an antioxidant for the skin, and it's the reason why you keep your skin healthy and radiant.

Avocados also contain antioxidants, carotenoids, and flavonoids that nourish skin that is dry and unhealthy. Avocado's nutrients help maintain clear skin.

Foods that can help reduce acne isn't just limited to the ones mentioned in this article. Apart from brown rice, broccoli, avocado, walnuts as well as green tea many other foods that may help to keep acne at bay.

Acne Triggers, Myths and More

Also, you should keep track of the foods which can cause acne. Be aware of your enemies. Find out what kinds of food items can cause acne.

Sugary Foods

Do you think that chocolate can cause acne? It's not the cacao -sugar is the culprit. A diet rich in fat and sugar could result in increased production of sebum, consequently, acne breakouts. Sugar also degrades elastin as well as collagen, proteins that help keep your skin soft, soft and soft and.

Sugary foods can also increase the blood sugar levels of your body and cause your body to release more insulin.

Some examples of foods that are sugary and could cause acne are candies such as chocolates, sodas and candies (but again it's the sugar that causes it that causes acne, so it's okay).

Greasy Foods

Don't blame it all on the grease. Eating grease-laden food like fries and burgers won't result in acne breakouts. The fat you consume isn't the same as the one that causes acne. If you rub your face with oily hands it could be a different story.

The risk of developing acne could even be more pronounced for those who work in an area that is frequently sprayed with grease e.g. flipping and frying Burgers. The air is full of oil particles that can clog your pores.

No, don't quit. Nothing is wrong with this type of job. It's not a reason to be embarrassed or intimidated by this type of job. Make sure you wash your face after returning back home in order to prevent breakouts.

Dairy Products

To be honest it's not been proven that there's a particular or specific connection between dairy products and acne. There is some evidence that suggests dairy products, specifically milk, can trigger breakouts of acne because of hormones in milk.

Certain studies, on the other hand, indicate that dairy foods can trigger an explosion of insulin in conjunction with sugary foods, this could result in more insulin being produced within the body.

Acne Myths

There are some myths that you've heard concerning acne and the facts about them. It's not always due to bad hygiene. The idea you're skin filthy could lead you to scrub or washing the face until the end, leading to more serious situations. It is possible that you will be left with irritated and inflamed skin.

* Don't press your pimples. Contrary to what some think, it doesn't let a blocked pore open. This will cause an increase in inflammation and increase the severity of acne.

* Acne could disappear in its own time, but it's not a problem in doing something about it, so it's a matter of ensuring that what you're doing doesn't cause more problems. There are treatments that you could consider that can not only address your acne issues but also avoid the occurrence of future acne issues.

It's not necessary to suffer the pain caused by acne. Look for treatments that can help clear pores and take swelling down. In the near future, your breakout will be gone in a flash.

Acne all the way to Extremes

Everyone is aware that prevention is superior to cure, however at times the actions you've taken aren't enough to prevent acne. In these situations the need for medication is to be addressed.

Don't worry about it however, as there are remedies that can help decrease the frequency of acne and also the chance of scarring.

Acne Treatments

If you have acne-related issues that aren't very extreme, you can opt to these medicines.

Salicylic Acid

Salicylic acid can be described as a white crystalline substance which aids in the breaking down of whiteheads and blackheads. It aids in the process of cell removal. It's a beta-hydroxyl acid (BHA) which doesn't just aid in removing pores, but also promotes the development in new cells.

Salicylic acid can be found in various products, including lotions, pads and creams and is often used as an Fungicide. It also helps to reduce swelling and inflammation.

Salicylic acids will only be felt while you are using it. The removal of its use will end the effects it has on the skin.

Resorcinol

Resorcinol is an encapsulated phenol that works in breaking down hardened rough and scaly skin. It assists in treating acne by getting rid of dead skin cells and combats infections by cleansing your skin.

Acne products typically contain sulfur mixed with resorcinol and can be used like a substitute for benzoyl Peroxide when treating skin that is sensitive. In addition to acne, resorcinol can also treat eczema, dandruff, eczema and other skin disorders.

Sulfur

Sulfur can be described as a yellow, crystalline solid that's used to treat skin disorders like eczema, psoriasis and acne. It's an over-the counter medication that aids in the breakdown of whiteheads and blackheads.

Sulfur must be mixed with other elements due to its unpleasant smell. There's no definitive solution yet to the question of the way sulfur can be used to treat acne, but it's been proven that sulfur oxidizes to create sulfuric acid with antibacterial properties.

Benzoyl Peroxide

Benzoyl peroxide can be described as a clear crystal substance that functions to bleach the skin as well as for treating moderate to mild instances of acne. It can also help eliminate acne-causing bacteria, known as Propionibacteria acnes, and reduce the glands producing oil.

It is also possible to use benzoyl peroxide to peel skin agent since it cleanses pores and removes dead skin cells. It comes in a variety of forms like creams, washes and lotions. Make sure you are cautious when using this product as it is not only bleaching fabrics but can also cause dry skin.

Acetone and Alcohol

Acetone helps in removing the skin's oily residues and alcohol acts as an antimicrobial, which reduces the amount of bacteria that cause skin infections.

They are commonly found in products for your skin, such as Astringents, cleaners, and toners particularly those designed suitable for those with oily skin. They aid in getting rid of excess oil from your skin and unblock your pores.

Cosmetic Procedures

Sometimes, you simply aren't able to take anymore, and are no longer able to be patiently waiting for the results of acne treatments and other natural treatments. In such cases, a variety of cosmetic treatments could be the best for your acne.

Chemical Peel

For a chemical peel powerful chemicals are employed to strip the skin's upper layer. This can smooth out any acne scars that are depressed and to smooth the appearance of the skin.

Chemical peels are a great option for dealing with acne-related scars which are small and subdued. The procedure performed by the surgeon is apply the chemical on the skin with a cotton-tipped applicator. The surgeon begins with the forehead, and then move up to the cheeks and then down to the chin.

Different kinds of chemicals can be utilized, based on the depth of the peel. Peels that are light won't need any healing time, whereas deep peels can require as long as two weeks of healing.

Dermabrasion

Dermabrasion utilizes either a burr fraise (diamond wheel with the rough edge) or a wire brush to remove away the top layer of the skin.

In the process of dermabrasion, the brush or burr rotates quickly, then takes off and evens out the skin's top layer. The process can inflict wounds on the skin, causing the skin to leak. The wounds heal and new skin cells will develop to replace the skin that was removed.

Laser Treatments

The superficial scars caused by acne are easily removed with laser treatments. Lasers will evaporate the top layer of skin and allow the new skin cells to form and expand.

The most commonly used methods of removing acne are the erbium YAG laser and pulsed yellow light laser with dye as well as ultrapulsed CO2 laser.

These procedures are usually performed in a surgeon's clinic or an outpatient department.

Similar to any other surgical procedure there is a chance of mild swelling, bruising and a little pain treatment for acne. You'll receive medicines to manage any discomfort.

Strategies to prevent Acne

"Prevention is always better than cure." Perhaps you have the money to cover all the medicines and treatments required to treat acne, but wouldn't it be better not to have anything to treat and enjoy healthy skin instead?

A healthy diet and an effective routine for beauty can be a huge help in treating and preventing acne, however, you'll get more benefits by incorporating lifestyle changes to fight against acne.

What can you do to avoid acne? Find out more here.

Drink water

Don't be afraid of drinking water. Drinking water has a myriad of health benefits to your body, including eliminating your body's waste and flushing out all the toxins out of the body and replenishing your body from within.

Toxins build up inside your body when your diet isn't sufficient with fluids. Your body's reaction is to flush out the toxins through your skin and lungs and, consequently, acne.

Your skin's health is affected by the food you consume. Since it is the biggest organ of the body that is responsible for regulating your body's temperature, it's important to maintain hydration. Drink plenty of water to keep it hydrated whatever the weather. A glass of water a day is perfect for your body, however you can take a drink with water like watermelons and grapes to hydrate.

There are many most effective skin products on the market however, you cannot beat the results of pure water for your skin.

Don't forget your sunscreen.

Do you think you don't require sunscreen? Consider reconsidering your position. Perhaps you don't notice the immediately the effects of sun's rays to the skin. However, if not vigilant sunburn can cause acne to get worse and eventually leave you suffering from dark marks. Additionally, being in the sun could increase the risk of skin cancer.

Another tip: go through all the ingredients listed and make sure that it does not contain any ingredient that can cause acne. Otherwise, all your efforts will be a go to. Make sure you choose non-comedogenic items; these products will not clog your pores.

Rest comfortably

"Sleeping well" sounds like the usual advice that you hear to prevent acne However an adequate night's sleep more like 7 hours per day will do to improve your skin.

While you sleep your body repairs the damage it went through throughout the previous day. This is why it's important to get enough sleepin this way your body will have enough time to repair its own problems.

A lack of sleep can easily cause stress, therefore you'll be more susceptible of getting acne. It's likely that you've heard about "beauty sleeping" and how more sleep improves your appearance and makes you appear more attractive.

Exercise

Apart from aiding you in losing those extra pounds, exercising and adhering to an exercise routine will aid in preventing acne.

Sweating helps eliminate toxins from your skin, which leads to a healthier and clearer skin. Additionally, you'll experience improved blood circulation, which removes the waste material on your skin. It also is able to bring oxygen into. Additionally, sweating can relax your body and helps take all the tension away.

Since sweat causes acne, be sure to remove sweat that has accumulated during your workout routine and try to shower as soon as you finish your workout.

Limit alcohol intake.

Alcohol is the main reason for acne, and regardless of whether you are a fan or not, you need to be careful with your alcohol consumption in order to avoid getting it to appear on your face.

Alcohol is harmful to your health because it alters the hormone levels. You've also learned that hormonal imbalances can lead to acne, so be careful not to push it.

Other indirect effects that alcohol has, for instance, it is linked to stress, which can cause acne. Alcohol can also impact the liver which is responsible for maintaining your skin's clear. It also can decrease the amount of water in your body and also shrink the pores of your skin.

That's it you're done with alcohol. maybe less drinks for you.

Chapter 17: Characteristics And Symptoms Of Acne

The most common signs of acne are an increase in the production of oily sebum on your skin. Microcomedones nodules, comedones pustules, scarring and pimples. But, the color of your skin is a factor that affects the appearance of acne.

Scars

Acne scars result from inflammation of the dermal layer skin. It affects about all people suffering from acne. The acne scars are due to the irregular healing caused by inflammation of the dermal layer. It is more likely that one will develop scars when acne is very severe, however, it could occur with any type of acne.

Acne scars that are atrophic are the most commonly seen type of acne scars . They are further classified into boxescar scars, icepick scars as well as rolling marks. The scars of ice-picks are very narrow, while deep scars stretch to the dermis. Boxcar scars are round with sharp edges while rolling scars are larger than scars from boxcar and icepick and are distinguished by a wave-like pattern that appears on the skin.

On the other hand hypertrophic scars are uncommon. They are firm and apex above the skin. They also stay within the original boundaries of the wound. Keloid scars can cause scar tissue that extends beyond the borders. Keloid scars occur more frequently when people have darker skin tones and can be seen on the body's trunk.

Pigmentation

It is caused by lesion of the skin called nodulae. These lesions can cause the dark spots and inflammation after the acne lesion is been healed. The inflammation stimulates melanocytes to make more melanin, which causes the skin to become dark.

The causes of acne

Beyond genes, the real triggers aren't well researched. Other possible triggers include food, hormones, infection, and stress. It is important to note that sunlight and cleanliness aren't in any way connected to acne.

Genes

The risk of developing acne is confirmed by studies regarding the prevalence of acne in twins as well as first cousins. In addition, the severity of acne may be linked with the XYY syndrome.

Hormones

Hormonal changes that occur during puberty and menses are also factors that can cause acne. As puberty progresses androgens are elevated, they directly contribute to the appearance of acne.

Infections

It is generally believed that an anaerobic strain of bacteria is responsible for acne, though the cause isn't as apparent.

Diet

There isn't a clear link between diet and acne. The diets with a high glycemic load are discovered to have an impact on the degree of acne. Additionally, numerous random studies have shown that diets with a lower levels of glycemic are capable of lessening acne. Furthermore, there is a lack of evidence that suggests that the dairy milk consumption is associated with a greater incidence and the severity of acne.

But, it's an established fact that milk has components that help in an increase in the amount of testosterone which are associated with acne.

Stress

Although the connection between stress and acne has been a topic of debate, there have been studies suggesting that a higher severity of acne is linked with stress levels that are high.

Environmental factors

Obstruction of the skin follicles by helmets or chinstraps could cause more irritation to acne already present.

Treatment and Management

There are many solutions for acne. They are believed to be effective in four ways: reducing inflammation, hormone regulation, eliminating P.acnes and normalizing the shedding of skin and also the production of sebum within the pores, which helps to prevent obstruction. A few of the most commonly used treatments are topical treatments like antibiotics, benzoyl peroxide , Retinoids, as well as systematic treatments which include hormonal gents , as well as oral Retinoids.

Benzoyl peroxide

It is a first-line treatment for moderate and mild acne due to its effectiveness and minor negative side effects, such as irritation to the skin. The drug kills P.acnes by making its proteins oxidized through the production by oxygen-free radicals as well as benzoic acid. Additionally, it can also be efficient in breaking down comedones, and in preventing inflammation. Bennzoyl can be combined with an oral antibiotic or Retinoids.

The adverse effects of this drug include skin photosensitivity dryness, redness, dryness and possibly peeling. The use of sunscreen is suggested to protect against sunburn. Be aware that excessive use of this can cause more breakouts.

Retinoids

They are medicines that lower inflammation, improve the cycle of life of hair follicles and lower the Sebum production. Retinoids stop the formation of skin cells which can cause obstruction in the hair follicle. It is the first treatment for acne, especially for people with dark skin. The most common topical retinoids comprise retinol, isotretinoin and adapalene. and the tazarotene.

Most of the time they can trigger an outbreak of acne, as well as facial flushing, which is far from irritation to the skin. This is due to the skin's sensitivity and are recommended to use them at night. Of all the retinoids Tretinoin is the most affordable however it is the most irritating. Adapalene can be the most soothing, but more expensive.

Antibiotics

They are commonly used in acne treatment, but they are getting less efficient. Antibiotics are typically used to treat moderate to moderately severe acne.

Hormonal agents

For females, it can be improved with all of the birth hormone control pills. They work by cutting down testosterone hormones produced in the ovaries. This results in a decrease in sebum production. This also helps reduce acne.

Azelaic acid

It has been demonstrated to be effective in treating mild to moderate pimples when it is applied to the skin. For best results, apply twice every throughout the day for 6 months. This treatment is extremely effective due to its capability to minimize the formation of skin cells within the hair follicle. In addition, it comes with anti-inflammatory and antibacterial properties. It also is able to reduce the appearance of skin and is great for post-inflammatory hyperpigmentation as well.

Salicylic acid

Salicylic acid blocks the reproduction of bacteria. It clears the pores in the skin, and stimulates removal of skin cells. The most common side effect of this treatment is dry and drier skin for people with darker skin.

Home remedies for acne

The skin is a vital organ within your body, so you must take it care of with the highest treatment you can get.

* Use apple cider vinegar

This is highly effective for acne since it kills bacteria. It also balances the skin's PH which makes it more difficult for bacteria to grow. Furthermore, it's astringent. assists in drying out of the excess oil in your face.

You'll need unfiltered and Apple cider vinegar that is pure, as well as clean water. Directions: Cleanse your face in water, then wipe it dry. Make use of one tablespoon of vinegar mixed with three parts water, put cotton wool in the vinegar, and then apply it directly on the affected area. Allow it to sit for at minimum ten minutes, or perhaps all the way through the night. It is possible to apply it multiple times during the day. Make sure you are cleanse your face following every application. Don't forget to apply a moisturizer when your skin is feeling dry.

* Honey, cinnamon and Cinnamon

Cinnamon is antimicrobial and assists in stopping the growth of bacteria. honey is an effective natural antibiotic. It is required two teaspoons of honey one teaspoon of cinnamon, and some paper towels.

Directions: wash your face, then pat it dry. Mix 2 teaspoons of honey and 1 teaspoon of cinnamon into an emulsion. Apply it to your face, and let it sit for about a quarter of an hour. Rinse clean and then dry the face. Paper towels can be used ideal for cleaning due to its sticky properties.

* Yogurt and milk

While it is true that dairy products can cause acne, applying milk topically can enhance your skin tone. The reason why it's believed that milk can cause acne is due to the hormones it contains and, as long as you don't drink it you're in good hands. Milk can be soothing on the skin that is irritated. In addition to milk, you could also make use of yogurt. The acids in it are antibacterial and the fat is moist. You need one tablespoon of plain, low-fat and full-fat yogurt milk, as well as one tablespoon of raw natural honey.

Directions: Mix one tablespoon of yogurt or milk and honey. Spread the mixture on the floor, allowing the first layer dry before applying the next. It should remain for around a quarter hour. Clean it off using the face towel to gently scrub your face in a circular manner and remove dead skin. Once you're done applying moisturizer.

* Egg whites

They're great for treating acne because they have vitamin A and proteins that aid in regenerating skin cells. They also absorb excess sebum, thereby eliminating the bacteria. It is necessary to have three eggs whites separated from yolks along with a bowl and a facial towel.

Directions: Rinse your face in water and rub it dry. Separate the yolks and whites. Mix the whites until they become foamy, then let them sit for a couple of minutes, apply it to your face and you concentrate on the areas that are affected. Be sure the first layer is dry before applying the next. Allow the mask to dry for at least 20 minutes prior to washing it out with hot water. Then wipe dry using an enveloping face towel. Apply moisturizer.

* Papaya

It eliminates dead skin cells as well as excess fats off the skin's surface leaving it soft and smooth. Papaya also contains an enzyme that decreases inflammation and helps in the treatment of pus.

Instructions: Wash your face with water and then pat dry. Mash the papaya until it's easy to apply it. Let it sit for about around a quarter of an hr after which you can rinse it using warm water. Apply a moisturizer as needed.

* Orange peel paste

Acne is the result of bacteria, along with dead skin cells and oil that block hair follicles. Oranges contain vitamin C as well as citric acid. They hinder reproduction of bacteria as well as the development in new cell. Take two orange peels and clear water.

Instructions: Wash your face in water and wipe it dry. Make a paste of the orange peels using the mortar and pestle or blender. Add water to it to make an even paste. Make sure that it's not overly thin. Apply the paste to your face or areas that are affected. Allow it to sit for 20 minutes, then rinse with water, dry and apply the moisturizer.

Tea tree oil

This is an agent that removes excess sebum as well as dead cells of the skin, thus clearing the pores. Furthermore, it has antibacterial properties that eliminate acne-causing bacteria. It should be dilute prior to use, and you should not ingest it.

You'll need a bottle tree oil, water that is clean as well as cotton wool.

Instructions: Wash your face thoroughly and then dry it. Mix one portion of tree oil and nine parts of water. A cotton ball is dipped into the mix and apply it to the areas affected. If you want you want to dilute the oil using aloe vera gel instead of water.

Honey and strawberries

Strawberries are a rich source of salicylic acid that is a key ingredient in various acne treatments as it unblocks pores as well as neutralizes the effects of bacteria. In addition, it shrinks the pores, preventing them from blocking and stimulating the development of new cells. However honey is an excellent anti-bacterial and anti-inflammatory ingredient. Two strawberries are required as well as two tablespoons honey in raw form.

Instructions: Wash your face with water, then dry. Wash the strawberries and then mash them thoroughly. Add the strawberries to 2 teaspoons of honey and mix it all together. Apply the cream to your face and allow it to remain for about 20 minutes before letting it rinse off with warm water. Dry and moisturise. The mixture is suitable for use twice per every week for a period of 30 days.

* Banana peel

The banana peels contain lutein, an antioxidant with a potent effect that decreases swelling, inflammation and encourages healthy development of cells. Therefore, the peelings can help reduce the appearance of redness.

Instructions: In circular motion, rub the peel over your face. Allow it to sit for about one hour, then wash.

* Aloe Vera gel

While it isn't soothing, it reduces swelling and the appearance of redness. Additionally, it has antibacterial properties. Cleanse your face, then apply it directly on the areas affected.

* Sodium bicarbonate

It is an antiseptic with the power to fight bacteria, fungus and eliminate excess oil. It also exfoliates the skin, leaving it soft and radiant. For a face masque, combine equal proportions in baking soda with water until you have a thick , thick paste. With circular movements massage your face with the paste for 2 minutes. Allow it to sit for a quarter of an hour and then rinse. Dry and apply a moisturizer.

If you wish to use it for scrub, mix half a cup baking soda and 12 cup water. Apply the paste on your face, massaging it thoroughly. After five minutes, wash using warm water. then dry and then moisturize.

* Lemon juice

This is a great way to eliminate breakouts due to of vitamins C and the citric acid. Additionally, it's an astringent which dries out redness and spots. Cleanse the lemon juice before heading out in the sunshine. You will need lemon juice as well as yogurt, and cotton wool. Wash your face thoroughly and dry. Apply lemon juice, in case it hurts too much Mix it with a little of yogurt.

* Steaming

Steam can reduce acne by unblocking pores and rid of the impurities on the skin. Bring a pot of water to a boil and then pour it into the bowl of a large size. Cool for a few minutes time before placing your face over the bowl and then cover it with an oversized towel that will steam. Remove the towel within 15 minutes and then dry. It is possible to do this at least every day or as often as you need. Be sure to moisturize when your pores have cleansed and opened.

* Garlic

It is a natural antibacterial agent. It is edible or apply it topically to lessen the severity of breakouts. If you can, extract the juice from the garlic, or crush it and mix in water. Never apply the juice on the skin, without diluting. Make use of your cotton wool for soaking the garlic or juice in water for approximately 10 minutes before covering the areas affected.

* Oatmeal

You can cook or soak oatmeal and use it as a mask for reducing inflammation and the redness. Prepare oatmeal , then add honey. Apply the oatmeal to the skin, let it sit for 30 minutes, after which you can wash it off with warm water.

* Sugar scrub

Sugar helps get rid of the excess skin cells that can block your pores through exfoliation. Combine sugar with honey olive oil or water , and you'll get a wonderful scrub that will heal your acne. It will take 1 1/2 cup of sugar white, the same amount for brown sugar 2 teaspoons coarse salt as well as half a cup of extra-virgin olive oil 10 tablespoons of pure vanilla extract, and 1 vanilla bean.

Instructions: Mix the white and brown sugar together with sea salt. Remove the caviar from the vanilla and incorporate it too. Pour 2 cups of the mixture into a measuring cup and then pack it into a neat. Add the oil extra-virgin on the top, and allow it to absorb into the mixture. It will form a layer over the over.

Mix it all up and add it to the remaining sugar, vanilla and salt mix. Add four tablespoons of vanilla extract, and incorporate it into the mix. Now you can keep your scrub in containers and then store.

* Avocado and honey

There are reports of breakouts caused by avocado due to the high fat content. But, there isn't any tangible evidence to support this assertion. Avocado is full of nutrients and vitamins that can help reduce the appearance of acne.

Instructions: Wash your face with water and pat dry. Remove the seeds from the avocado, then mash it. Mix it together with honey till it becomes an oil. Then apply it to the skin and let it sit for half an hour. After this, wash your facial area with warm, clean water. dry and then moisturize.

Keep your pillowcase clean and bed sheets tidy

The pillowcase should be washed and sheets at a minimum every week. Cleaning your pillowcase will help prevent breakouts.

Do not touch your face.

Beware of the itching and peeling, scratching or rub your skin. Beware of touching the face at all times. Your hands contain huge amounts of oil and bacteria derived from objects that you've had contact with. If you must contact your face, you should utilize the back of your hand, which has been in lesser contact with foreign contact. If you are suffering from acne, you should avoid the temptation to rub it to ensure quick healing.

* Keep your minty fresh by adding mint

Mint contains menthol, which acts as a painkiller and as an anti-inflammatory. It can help swelling fade as well as ease the discomfort that is caused by swelling.

Instructions: Wash your face with water and then dry. Smash the leaves and apply them to your face and allow them to sit for

10 minutes before washing away with cool water.

Acne myths

A lot of people are misinformed regarding this issue due to conflicting facts. But, if you understand the truth from the truths, you can determine the best method to take care of your skin.

* Dirty skin can cause acne.

It's impossible to be further from the reality. Acne is not because of dirty or unclean habits. Be cautious not to scrub your skin too often with harsh soaps since this can cause more damage to the skin. It is best to be gentle when it comes to cleaning your skin.

* Chocolate and easy foods

The results have shown that they produce little or no impact whatsoever on acne. The food you consume has an effect, for instance dairy products and carbohydrates raise blood sugar levels, or may contain hormones that cause acne, but that's not all the time.

* Stress

Theoretically speaking, stress influences hormones, which can cause acne. But, lots of suffer from stress. If stress is the real reason behind it for acne, how many people would have acne?

* No moisturizer is recommended for people who suffer from acne.

Moisturizers can help balance your skin and ensuring that there isn't any excess oil.

* Sunlight can eliminate acne

This isn't the solution.

Tips to prevent acne

Make sure you keep your face fresh

It is suggested to cleanse the face two times every day to eliminate impurities dead skin cells, dead skin cells, and oily residue. Cleanse your face using warm water and mild cleanser. In addition, be careful not to rub your skin too hard by gently washing it with an ointment-like cloth or hands.

Also, make sure to rinse thoroughly and then dab dry using an untidy face towel.

* Use a moisturizer

Many of the products used for the treatment of acne contain ingredients that can leave your skin dry. So ensure that you use an oil-based moisturizer. Pick a moisturizer suitable for your skin type, dry or oily.

Try an over-the-counter acne treatment

Acne products need no prescription. However, you must apply these products with care and according to the directions.

• Reduce the amount of makeup you apply.

If you're experiencing an acne breakout, do not apply any makeup or if you need to, be sure to remove it by the time you're done.

* Exercise and diet

Drink plenty of fluids to stay hydrated, as this will aid you in maintaining a healthy and beautiful skin. Doctors have also recognized that diet plays an important part in the development of acne. A balanced diet can help your body combat acne. Exercise is essential for the reduction of acne because it reduces the amount of stress your body experiences. If

you exercise, make sure to shower and clean up right following. A lot of sweat on the body can cause bacteria to grow and the problematic areas to appear.
Avoid drinking excessively or smoking
Studies have linked the presence of toxins in alcohol and tobacco to acne.

Conclusion

In the end the acne issue is a multifaceted issue that requires a comprehensive solution. Making permanent, healthy modifications to your life is the only way you can have be truly healthy and have healthy skin. My suggestion is to make wise choices regarding the way you spend your time, what you make, as well as your food choices.

If you commit yourself to lead a healthier life now , you'll benefit in the future. Actually, I believe it's the best present you can give yourself! In that regard, I encourage you to get involved. Don't just read the book, but follow its instructions. It's about long-term health choices in your life. Make this a priority for yourself!

www.ingramcontent.com/pod-product-compliance
Lightning Source LLC
Chambersburg PA
CBHW050235120526
44590CB00016B/2101